Joseph Kidd

The laws of therapeutics

or, The science and art of medicine

Joseph Kidd

The laws of therapeutics
or, The science and art of medicine

ISBN/EAN: 9783742815668

Manufactured in Europe, USA, Canada, Australia, Japa

Cover: Foto ©Lupo / pixelio.de

Manufactured and distributed by brebook publishing software
(www.brebook.com)

Joseph Kidd

The laws of therapeutics

CONTENTS.

THE LAWS

OF

THERAPEUTICS.

We must be content to stand before nature and ask questions. Nature is only to be subdued by submission.—BACON.

CHAPTER I.

HISTORICAL.

In the following pages I desire to make a fresh and unbiassed inquiry into the fundamental principles of the science and art of healing, to ascertain if medicine can be brought into the position of an exact science, or if it is to remain merely an art.

I have endeavored to forget men and their systems, and to search for truth—for all truth. The true student of nature ever delights to lay self aside, to present his offering to the growth of knowledge and withdraw, that God and His truth may be all in all.

Of all the studies that of therapeutics, or the treatment of disease, ought to be the most accurate. With human life at stake, it saddens the heart to think that chance should rule where law ought to reign. The

2

life of a human being, or the usefulness of a vital
organ such as the heart or brain, may depend upon
accuracy in the application of curative measures. The
physician should endeavor to ascertain if the good
providence of God has ordained exact laws for the
selection of curative agents in the treatment of disease.
If such laws exist, how solemn the position of those
who would reject them.

The most pressing question at the present time for
the physician to ascertain is, whether the treatment of
disease is to depend on mere opinion, which varies
with each doctor and perishes with the individual, or
on laws which, founded on the immutable truth of facts,
can never perish but must endure through all ages?

Medicine is yet to a great extent a mere collection
of facts and of opinions which vary from year to year
according to the theories of the most prominent men.
Thus, the practice of physicians thirty years ago is at
present regarded as worse than useless; whereas, had
law governed their practice, all truth in that practice
would have remained as the inheritance of science, and
available for their successors: truth can never perish.

*Nothing can be more repugnant to an ordinary mind
than the thorough sifting of deepseated, long-familiar-
ized notions.**

The discoveries in physiology, pathology, and the
art of medicine, during the past thirty years, have been
great and most beneficial, but that the *practice* of therapeutics is not an exact *science* founded upon definite
principles is but too plain.   Witness the words of Sir

---

* Grote's Plato, vol. ii, p. 12.

Thomas Watson, in 1869, to the Clinical Society: "It seems to have been thought in some quarters that I had renounced my faith in physic, that I undervalued the resources and usefulness of our art. Such a notion is the very reverse of the truth. I am anxious to have the effects of remedies carefully ascertained and certified, just because I have so great faith in their real force. What I deprecate, what I fain would see altered, what it is one great end of this society to do away with— is the vagueness of aim, the uncertainty of result, the merely tentative nature of too many of our prescriptions.

"Far from thinking that our warfare with disease is a vain warfare, I am only desirous that our arms should have the precision of the modern rifle instead of the wild flight of the old-fashioned smooth-bore. Probably I have even greater reliance than many physicians on the virtues of drugs, of what used to be called simples—a word I like, because it helps continually to suggest to one's mind the golden rules that their administration should be simple, that they should be mixed as little as possible with other substances which might confuse or vitiate the conclusions to be drawn from their actual operation."

The testimony of Brown-Séquard is equally significant: "We find very little is known as regards the real and ultimate mode of action of remedies. This is much to be lamented, as therapeutics will cease to be empirical only when this last kind of knowledge shall be fully obtained." *

The study of therapeutics includes all that concerns

---

* Brown-Séquard, Lancet, March 10th, 1866.

the prevention and treatment of disease, the knowledge and use of medicines, food, drink, baths, exercise, gymnastics, electricity, galvanism; it also includes all surgical applications. In order to understand the exact state of therapeutics now, it will be necessary to take a rapid view of the varied phases of medical practice from the earliest ages to the present time.

In sketching out the leading features of therapeutics, it is necessary for our purpose to pass over much ordinary history of medicine, except what concerns the treatment of disease.

In the most ancient history of medicine—Egyptian, Persian, and Grecian—we find that the pursuit of astrology and magic was so intimately mixed up with the practice of medicine, that all their early records are vague and untrustworthy.

In the early ages of the world the tide of civilization flowed from East to West. Thus the most ancient records are Egyptian. Even the oldest medical traditions of the Greeks are traceable to the Egyptians. The Egyptian Isis and Hermes may be regarded as the prototypes of Apollo and Mercury.

"The extreme antiquity of medical science in Egypt may be inferred from the fact that the medical papyrus at Berlin, fourteenth century B.C., contains the copy of a treatise on inflammation (onchet) which was found 'written in ancient writing, rolled up in a coffer under the feet of an Anubis in the town of Sokhem (Letopolis), in the time of His Sacred Majesty Thot the Righteous. After his death it was handed on to King Suat on account of its importance. It was then restored to its place under the feet of the statue, and sealed up by the sacred scribe and wise chief of the physicians.'

"In Egypt, about the eleventh century B.C., there was a college of physicians, who belonged to the sacerdotal class. They were not confined to one sex. The sculptures confirm Exodus i. 15, that women practiced medicine."

"Medical science attained so high a degree of perfection in Egypt that there were specialists in the different branches of the art, and the physician was only allowed to practice in his own branch. There were oculists and dentists, those who treated mental disorders and those who investigated obscure diseases, οἱ δὲ τῶν ἀφανεῶν νούσων. There are medical papyri which treat of these several diseases. In the Hermaic books a whole chapter is devoted to diseases of the eye, and mummies have been found in Thebes with their teeth stopped in gold." *

To guard the people against quacks and the rash experiments of young doctors, the Egyptian physicians were required to follow the rules laid down in the medical treatises preserved in the principal temple of each city; the idea being that the old must be better than the new. Aristotle, however, says that they were allowed to alter the orthodox treatment; yet if they did so it was at their peril, as their own lives were forfeit for the life of the patient.

The Babylonians and Assyrians alone, among the great nations of antiquity, had no physicians. The

---

* Westminster Review, No. 104, p. 430.

sick man was laid on a couch in the public square,
and the passers-by were required to ask him the nature
of his disease, so that if they or any of their acquaint-
ances had been similarly afflicted they might advise
him as to the remedies he should adopt.*

" Æsculapius, to some historians a mythical person-
age, appears in human form at Epidaurus, and extends
his saving right hand over all the earth, to heal the
souls that are in error and the bodies that are diseased."
His treatment was so successful that after his death
festivals called Asclepia were celebrated to his memory
at Athens and many other parts of Greece. Temples
for the treatment of the sick, called Asclepiades, were
founded in honor of him. They were generally built
in the most healthy places that could be chosen, and
ornamented with votive tablets, on which were in-
scribed the diseases which had been successfully treated
and the remedies employed. The *Asclepiades* placed†
their chief reliance on hygienic means—baths, open-
air exercise, and moderation in food and drink. The
Asclepiades meddled not with the dead ; by their laws
no one was allowed to die in the establishment.

Hippocrates, whose genius reigned without a rival
for twenty-three centuries, was nurtured in the famous

* Westminster Review, No. 104, p. 428.

† The Asclepias, or the therapeutic establishment, presented
singular advantages; generally built on some healthily elevated
spot, or near a mineral spring, with a doctor presiding over all
its arrangements. The patient was put through a preparatory
course of treatment by baths, careful dieting, perfect quiet, for
a week before the real medicinal treatment commenced.

Asclepias of Cos. He was born 460 B.C., and was one of a family whose members had practiced medicine for three centuries in the temple of Cos. In addition to his own vast experience, he used freely the materials of the tablets or archives preserved by his family in the temple.

Medical science owes much to his accurate observation of the natural history of disease. In therapeutics, however, he fell into the cardinal mistake of regarding disease as a positive entity or substance, not a derangement of health. Hippocrates inveighed with great warmth against all those who corrupted medicine by introducing vague hypotheses; yet he lost sight of his own teaching, and based his treatment, not on the distinct facts of relationship between the action of medicine on the healthy organism and on the diseased, but upon his own opinion of the cause of disease. Yet he caught a glimpse of the truth, although it did not much influence his teaching.

"Law rules all things," he writes; and yet he is one of the first to leave facts, the only true foundation of law, for the fanciful theories of his own imagination. Hence, much as he enriched the knowledge of the origin, natural course, and termination of disease, he did but little for the science of therapeutics.

Like the best physicians of all ages, Hippocrates excelled in prognosis, owing to his sagacity in observing the natural history of disease. Hippocrates was the first to acknowledge the principles of nature ($\varphi \acute{v} \sigma \iota \varsigma$) in superintending and regulating the bodily functions. With Socrates and Plato for contemporaries, his writings owe much to the speculative philosophy of those great men. Looking upon the disease as something foreign to the human body,* he treated, not the individual sick person, but his own idea of the disease. He viewed disease as an excess of blood in spring, of yellow bile in summer, of black bile in autumn, and of phlegm in winter. He used medicines according to his opinion of their nature, not according to the relationship between their action and the disease. The primary pathological doctrine of Hippocrates was that of the "Humoral Pathology"—that the essential seat of disease was in the fluids of the body. The belief in "nature" as a presiding principle naturally led to the teaching of the "restorative power of nature" in the removal of disease.

He regarded the body as composed of the four primary elements, air, fire, earth, water, variously combined to produce the four cardinal humors, blood, phlegm, bile, and black bile; to the equipoise of which he attributed health, and to the loss of such balance disease.† His chief practice was depletion, either by the lancet, or by purgatives or expectorants. Hippocrates had the innate genius of the true physician, and was far wiser in the treatment of disease than his system would indicate. With the essential doctrine of treat-

* Yet when Socrates, the one whose wisdom it ever was to reduce all mental phenomena to their ultimate elements, and natural things to their most simple forms, was asked how he would define disease, he answered: "A disarrangement of the body."

† History of Medicine, Dr. Meryon, p. 23.

ment founded on his idea of the nature of disease and of the nature of the action of medicines, he was yet in reality the founder of the rational empirical method. He adopted remedies not in relation to his system but which seemed in any way useful in disease—*ex usu in morbis.* The " practice of Hippocrates may be defined as a rational empiricism."

Hippocrates lived in an age in which intolerance was not active, hence the rapid progress of medicine during his life. In Galen's time the dogma of authority flourished, which, in the words of Dr. Lefort, of Paris, "immobilized" science; liberty favored its advance.*

The first well-marked schism in medicine, about 250 B.C., arose from the mistake of Hippocrates in leaving the region of pure observation† for that of speculation, as a natural reaction from which arose the sect of the Empirics, priding itself on following experience alone, to the neglect of anatomy and physiology, because they savored of "rationalism," and all but repudiating etiology and diagnosis. Against this came a strong protest in the sect of the Dogmatists, claiming all authority for doctrine or theory.

From the speculations and discords of the Empirics

---

* Dr. Lefort, of Paris, Lancet, Nov. 22d, 1873, p. 757.

† " Facts alone have been employed to establish other natural sciences, whilst in medicine the human imagination has been taxed to the utmost in framing hypotheses to accord with, or account for, the various phenomena which are presenting themselves to the physician's notice."—The History of Medicine, by Dr. Meryon.

and Methodists in the early centuries, Greece was aroused to the stern reality of disease by the occurrence of the terrible pestilence at Athens in the year 430 B.C., so admirably described by Thucydides. Like most epidemics, it came through Egypt from Persia or Ethiopia. It first appeared at the Piræus, the seaport of Athens, where its advent was so virulent and sudden that popular report at once ascribed it to poison cast into the wells by the Peloponnesians.

The dry, healthy, elevated situations of many of the chief Greek cities rendered the occurrence of epidemics so rare that little heed was taken of them in Greece. But it was not so in ancient Rome ; the unwholesome situation of that great city was much aggravated by the overcrowding of men and animals in its narrow streets. The plague proved a deadly scourge to its inhabitants. Medical science had but very uncertain skill to investigate its cause, and scanty resources for its treatment. After so many outbreaks of epidemics, the need for drainage of the city was recognized. The "Cloaca Maxima" remains to this day as one of the most remarkable monuments of ancient Rome. Even at the present time it is astonishing to look upon its admirable masonry and the stream of clear water flowing through the ancient channel.

Gradually breaking away from the speculations and drugging of the Greeks, the Roman people took kindly to men called quacks, such as Asclepiades, the friend of Cicero. Dissatisfied with the drugging of that day, he treated his patients by hygienic means—careful dieting, baths, exercise, and change of habits of life.

He became the horror, the incarnation of evil to the "apothecaries" of his day; the men who then, as now, see good in nothing except mixtures, pills, plasters, and other manufactures of their craft. To discourage drugging and substitute wise regulation of habits of life, is still an unpardonable sin to the orthodox practitioner.

Weary with the quarrels of the Empirics and Dogmatists arose the sect of Eclectics, professing to select the good and avoid the bad in all the systems of the Empirics, Dogmatists, Methodists, etc. Of all the "sects" that of the Eclectics was about the worst. Eclecticism in medicine is like the mule in creation, essentially barren. The Eclectics enjoyed a short-lived existence, and soon made way for the "Skeptics," whose reign extended over most of the second century of the Christian era. They were satisfied to maintain "that nothing could be known and nothing demonstrated." To such crude nihilism Christianity came in as a resting-place. Till its doctrines became corrupted it proved the antidote of Skepticism. But, alas! corruption came early. In the second and following centuries, the monks and anchorites destroyed the simplicity of Christian faith and doctrine, and changed the truth into necromancy and charlatanism.

For six centuries, i. e., from Hippocrates to Galen, all is vague and contradictory in therapeutics till the latter introduced a very positive theory of medical practice. Galen was born at Pergamos, A.D. 131, and studied medicine at Alexandria at the time when all was conflict between the rivals sects of Dogmatists,

Empiries, Methodists, and Pneumatics. He endeavored to bring physicians back to nature and accurate observation, but he mixed up with this much speculation and many fanciful theories, in the attempt to follow the philosophy of Plato and Aristotle. For upwards of fifteen centuries his system reigned supreme in Europe. Whilst Hippocrates founded his treatment of disease on his own opinion of the nature of the *disease,* Galen* founded his system on his idea of the nature of *medicines,* regarding each to be either hot or cold, dry or moist, etc. He forsook the region of observation and facts for speculative opinions about the the nature of disease and the nature of medicines ; yet he indicated the necessity for seeing a relationship between the action of medicines on the human body in health and in disease: that relationship being of " con-

---

* " Galen, in the second century after Christ, did more for medicine than any ten men since. He fell upon evil times, when the old faiths had rotted away, and the old philosophies were found cold guides, when swinish debauchery was the only real enjoyment, and when those who cared not to live for that cared not to live at all. The physicians of his day at Rome were generally panders to vice, slaves ready to adopt any opinion most agreeable to their patrons, believing in nothing because everything seemed a sham. Yet, in the midst of the society of the doomed empire, Galen buckled himself to his life-work with a full faith that there was a true art of healing latent among the impostures he saw practiced around him. It would seem to be from Plato that he acquired the notion of diseases being additional forces, foreign and inimical to the animal, with a birth, prime, and decline, like those of a physiological nature. The whole duty of a physician, according to him, lay in opposing the action of these morbid forces (ἐναντίωσις). Remedies were

traria contrariis," or the Antipathic Law,* which for 1600 years has been associated with his name. He neglected to observe the exact symptoms of the action of medicines on the healthy, and unfortunately taught his followers to apply the law of "contraria contrariis" according to their opinion of the nature of disease and of the nature of the drug action.

This substitution of the doctor's opinion for the exact observation of facts has been the cause of the barren state of therapeutics since his time to the present age. It has borne bad fruit to science, having caused physicians for many centuries to neglect the observation of the actual phenomena of disease, and to substitute theory or opinion. To the present hour this is the deadly gap in the science of medicine. The action of each medicine on the healthy body is little understood; such knowledge is confused, the little that is known is muddled by the opinions of such and such a doctor that it is "alterative" or "sedative," or some other word that only serves to confuse knowledge.

Galen had a true idea of the first duty of the physician—to aim at maintaining the different organs of the body in their natural condition, and at re-establishing their healthy function when diseased. With the genius which enabled him to acquire an ascendency over all the physicians of his times, Galen was deficient in the accurate observation of disease which characterized Hip-

---

therefore to be sought which in a healthy man would produce symptoms contrary to those of the disease."—The Quarterly Review, No. 252, April, 1868, p. 538.

* History of Medicine, Dr. Meryon, p. 137.

pocrates. He was accused of cowardice for running
away from the plague. His practice was complicated
with speculative doctrines and fancies, which proved a
fertile source of dispute for many centuries.

From the time of Galen to the first incursion of the
Goths (in the fifth century after Christ), medical schools
flourished at Rome and Constantinople. The fierce
destructive energy of the Gothic invasion scattered medical science, and left it for many centuries in the hands
of monks and priests—the rulers of that dark age—
from the fifth to the eleventh century; during which,
in the words of Gibbon, "it would be difficult, within
the same historical space, to find more vice and less
virtue."

Through all the early Christian centuries, the priest-
hood monopolized the scanty knowledge of the times,
and exercised its power to impress the people with a
superstitious awe of their knowledge, which enabled
them to rule men's bodies as well as their minds.

The Asclepias, or hygienic establishment of the
Greeks, became gradually changed into the hospital,
over which the monks presided, and in which much
was done to alleviate the sufferings of the poor within
whose reach was the hospital near at hand. Few but
the rich could travel to the Asclepias, far away on some
favored hill.

As the Greeks received the idea of the " Asclepias "
from the Egyptian "dispensary," so Christianity took
the idea of the hospital from the Greek Asclepias, the
improvement upon the latter being so great as to be-
tray Dr. Farrar, in his *Life of Christ*, to exaggerate

not a little in writing, "Amidst all the boasted civilization of antiquity there existed no hospitals, no penitentiaries, no asylums." The true testimony to Christianity being that it found a partial imperfect asylum for the sick and the well-to-do, who could travel long distances to the Asclepias, and brought to the door of the poor an hospital where the weak, the necessitous, the sick, could find shelter and care "without money and without price."

The gross darkness of the Druids, amongst the Gauls and Britons, reproduced the heathen idolatry of the early Greek philosophy in ascribing diseases to the anger of the gods, to appease whom was the sacred privilege of the priests. "Numberless charms, spells, and incantations were made use of, to deceive the patient and increase their own consequence."

Little by little the practice of medicine passed from the hands of benevolent men trying to help the sick, into those of the impudent quack professing to understand the secrets of nature, and pretending to possess occult and supernatural means of cure, selling talismans and charms as preservatives against disease, changing the practice of medicine into mysticism and magic, too often for gain.

As medical knowledge declined in the West, after the first siege of Rome, A.D. 408, it flickered into a very feeble flame in the East and in Spain, during the reign of the Saracens, who lacked genius and devoted all their energy to a steady imitation of Galen, "the god of their idolatry." In their therapeutics a very large part is taken up with pretended specifics, charms,

talismans, amulets. Although they added many* articles to the Materia Medica, the treatment of disease
was but little advanced. To the Arabian physicians
medical science owes one great boon, the institution of
chemical laboratories. Geber's vain search after a
universal remedy was fruitful to science by instituting
the habit of chemical research. An offshoot of the
Arabian school flourished at Cordova in Spain (the
parent of the French school at Montpellier). The off-
spring of a degenerating race, it was rich in nothing
but in excerpta from Galen and Hippocrates. "They
borrowed so much that their writings were soon for-
gotten."

Rhazes was the most distinguished man of the school
of Cordova. The honesty and uprightness of his life
were the truest answer to the impostors and quacks of
that age. Another of the same school deserves notice,
Avicenna, of whom it is related that "whenever he
recognized a new truth in others, or discovered one
himself, he is said to have prostrated himself in humble
thankfulness to God."†

The vain search of the alchemists after the "philos-
opher's stone" was prosecuted with vigor in the thir-
teenth century. It was supposed—besides having the
property of producing gold—to possess the power of
curing all diseases, and hence obtained the title of the
"universal medicine." In its primary object the search

---

* "The Arabians added camphor, senna, musk, nux vomica,
aloes, manna, cassia, rhubarb, and tamarinds."—History of Medicine, by Dr. Meryon, p. 127.

† History of Medicine, by Dr. Meryon, p. 113.

of course failed, yet in the numerous efforts which the alchemists made to accomplish their object they acquired considerable information about the nature and properties of the substances employed by them in their researches.

Then arose the sect of Chemical Physicians, who opposed themselves to the Galenists. Amongst the most distinguished was Paracelsus, a man of the most consummate audacity and presumption. He boasted that he had discovered the "elixir vitae," the universal remedy of which mankind had been so long in search; but his own death, at the age of forty-eight, served to humble the confidence of his followers. The leading principle of the chemists was that the living body is subject to the same chemical laws as inanimate matter, and that all the phenomena of life may be explained by the operation of these laws. They asserted that disease was caused by an acid or alkaline humor. Their therapeutics were invariably "contraria contrariis" all through.*

In the sixteenth century rapid strides were made in anatomical investigation, amply rewarded in the discovery of the circulation of the blood by the immortal

---

* "Still, it can hardly be questioned that quite up to our own times the Galenical notion of curing diseases by their contraries has held its ground bravely. Its permanence has been in a great measure due to its openness to receive modifications and partial reform. One of the most important of these is an amplification of Hippocrates's suggestion, that diseases contain in themselves their own cure, into Sydenham's attribution of their phenomena *to an effort of nature to get rid of some noxious material*."—The Quarterly Review, No. 252. April, 1869.

Harvey, and of the absorbent system by Asselli, Rud-
sheck, and Bartholine, while the structure and office
of the lungs, and the relation which they bear to the
heart, were explained by Malpighi, Hooke, etc.

In 1659 the learned Englishman, Willis, published
his celebrated treatise on fermentation and fever, a
doctrine fashionable for a time, and again revived at
the present time. Willis was succeeded by Sydenham,
who, though his writings abound in theory, had the
great merit of not allowing his speculative opinions to
interfere with his treatment. In one important point
he agreed very nearly with Hippocrates, that diseased
action consists essentially in an effort of nature to
remove some morbid or noxious cause, and that the
great object of the practitioner is to assist in bringing
about the crisis, and to regulate the actions of the
system so as to prevent either their excess or defect.
Sydenham's idea of attributing the phenomena of disease to an effort of nature to get rid of some noxious
material, was the first real innovation or change from the
Galenical principle of "contraria contrariis curantur."

This practice consisted rather in attempts to palliate
certain symptoms than to counteract or remove their
cause. Sydenham's natural sagacity caused him to feel
the value of the inductive method, while unaware of
the great importance to the science of medicine of the
great truths which had been promulgated by Bacon.
Sydenham has been styled the English Hippocrates,
and his writings, whilst abounding in theory, resemble
those of Hippocrates in containing the most accurate
description of disease. His genius enabled him to

seize upon the most essential features of a disease, and to direct his attention to those points alone which tended to illustrate the nature of the morbid changes that were produced. His observations upon epidemic diseases possess special interest.

In the seventeenth century, Harvey, Malpighi, and Ruysch, imbued with the newly-discovered knowledge of the circulation of the blood, taught that the cause of disease was to be found in spasm and relaxation of the vessels, but, like all the doctrines founded on opinions and not on facts, the gain to therapeutics was very scanty.

In the seventeenth century, in Italy, Bonet laid the foundation of anatomical pathology. His work "Sepul-chretum" described a large number of cases of diseases, with their history, and the appearances observed upon dissection. His investigations were followed up by his illustrious pupil Morgagni. Morbid anatomy could only see disease in the solids or the fluids of the body, and expressed its therapeutics by free depletion, to get rid of the morbid matter from the blood; but in spite of all the bleeding, and contrary to the theory, the patients died so fast that physicians began to distrust the lancet. In Italy also arose the Mathematical School, inaugurated by Bonelli. He maintained that all the functions of the body may be explained by the application of the ordinary* physical laws—hydro-statics, hydraulics.

The doctrines of the chemical and mathematical

---

* This doctrine is again becoming fashionable with the modern school of advanced physiologists.

physicians were alike rejected by the celebrated Stahl, who was born at Anspach in 1660. He observed the action which the mind exercises over the body, and proved that these effects could not be referred merely to a chemical or mechanical agent. He bestowed all his attention on the study of what he termed vital actions, regarded it as the duty of the physician to superintend the action of the "anima;" generally, to co-operate with its efforts; if irregular or injurious, to endeavor to restrain or counteract them.

While Stahl and Hoffmann were promulgating their doctrines in the University of Halle, the celebrated Boerhaave was teaching at Leyden. He (Boerhaave) had a mind and character peculiarly well adapted for the age in which he lived, when a variety of new facts and hypotheses were brought into view, and when it required consummate judgment to weigh the opposing evidence. His great object in the formation of his system was to collect all that was valuable from preceding writers, and by means of these materials to erect a system which should be eclectic and true: "What may be called the eclectic state, trying all things with a candor and real love of improvement which gives the best omens of a still higher success."*

The grand error of Boerhaave was, like the besetting sin of so many, that he depended more upon opinions than upon facts. His system accordingly could not stand the test of experience in an age when an active spirit of investigation prevailed. It was generally discarded soon after the death of its originator.

---

* Carlyle on French Poetry; Voltaire, p. 45.

Haller, a pupil of Boerhaave, and contemporary of Cullen, has been termed the father of modern physiology.* Although not engaged in the practice of medicine, he contributed more to our knowledge of disease than any of his predecessors. His long and well-directed experimental researches established his theory of irritability and sensibility as specific properties attached to the two great systems of the animal frame, the muscular and nervous, to which, either separately or conjointly, he referred all the phenomena of the living body. Moreover, in addition to his actual discoveries, he rendered even a greater service to science by his example of abstaining from all mere speculative opinions, and by forming his deductions from experiment and facts.

From Hippocrates to Haller medical treatment was more or less dependent upon the *opinions* of the doctor as to the nature of medicines and disease.

"The laws of nature are not things which we can evolve by any speculative method. On the contrary, we have to discover them in the facts: we have to test them by repeated observation or experiment. In proportion only as they hold good under a constantly increasing change of conditions, in a constantly increasing number of cases, and in the greater delicacy in the means of observation, does our confidence in their trustworthiness rise."†

---

* Next to Haller, John Hunter, in England, gave its truest bent to human physiology by the careful study of comparative anatomy, which has borne rich fruit to humanity ever since.

† Helmholtz, Popular Lectures on Scientific Subjects, p. 370.

Haller, in the eighteenth century, was the first practically to teach that the true guide to the treatment of disease must be sought for in the accurate knowledge of the action of medicinal agents on the human body in health. "In the first place, the remedy is to be tried on the healthy body, without any foreign substance mixed with it; a small dose is to be taken, and attention is to be directed to every effect produced by it; for example on the pulse, the temperature, the respiration, the secretions. Having obtained their obvious phenomena in health, you may then pass on to experiment on the body in a state of disease."

The genius of Haller gave its impetus to the mind of Hahnemann, who labored for many years to elucidate the physiological action of medicinal agents, often with artificial and exaggerated minuteness. His great enthusiasm led him to reject *in toto* all that savored of Galen; caused him to ascribe too much power to medicinal substances, and to impute too little to the practical management of the patient's habits, diet, exercise, baths, external applications, choice of climate, soil, and situation.

Contemporary with Haller lived Hahnemann, born in 1755, at Meissen, near Dresden, where he settled in medical practice in 1784. Five years afterwards he removed to Leipsic. There, whilst engaged in translating Cullen's *Materia Medica* into German, meditating upon the action of cinchona bark in ague, he took large doses of it, to learn its action on the healthy body. In the course of four days he experienced the symptoms of ague. It then occurred to him that *the reason why cinchona cures ague* is because of the power inherent in it to *produce symptoms in a healthy person* similar to those of ague.

From this the system of Homœopathy became gradually evolved,* after many years of patient labor in proving, upon his own person, the qualities or actions of various medicines. Gradually also he began to lessen the amount of dose, not by any logical deduction from facts, but rather from an arbitrary conceit of his own fancy, till he broached the mystical doctrine of infinitesimal doses and of dynamization. The grand mistake of Hahnemann was, not to have rested in the promulgation of the primary law of therapeutics. In forsaking the accurate interpretation of facts, he became a "system builder," like Galen or Boerhaave—essentially a dogmatist, *i. e.*, one whose influence as a teacher depended largely upon the acceptance of his

---

* It is most interesting to notice that other observers at a distance corroborated this proving of cinchona, as evidenced by the following extract from Trousseau and Pidoux, Traité de Thérapeutique, etc., seventh edition, 1862:

" Each day's observations," says M. Bretonneau, " prove that cinchona, given in a large dose, determines in a great number of subjects a very marked febrile movement. The characters of this fever, and the time when it shows itself, vary in different individuals: oftenest tinnitus aurium, deafness, and a species of intoxication precede the invasion of this fever; a slight shivering then occurs; a dry heat, accompanied by headache, succeeds to these first symptons; they gradually abate, and end by sweat. Far from yielding to new and higher doses of this medicine, the fever produced by cinchona is only exasperated "

Commenting on this testimony of M. Bretonneau, who was in his day one of the most eminent of French physicians, MM. Trousseau and Pidoux continue:

fundamental doctrines or dogmata as regards the nature of disease, its causes, and its cure.*

The tendency of the present age is to mistrust the "systems" of medicine which rely upon doctrines or dogmata; to rely altogether on the accurate facts of experience searched out by the most perfect methods of investigation, proved at the bedside of the sick. Such facts, combined into laws by a true method of interpretation, become the fruitful source of blessing to humanity in its time of suffering.

With all his vast practice, it is singular that Hahnemann published the records of but two cases, one of which was a model of accurate description—a case of gastralgia, for which he prescribed the strongest or mother tincture of bryonia, which effectually cured the disease in a few days.

" Mrs. S., laundress, forty and odd years old, had been laid up for three weeks, when she consulted me, on September 1st, 1815.

" 1. At every movement, especially when treading, she has stitches in the pit of her stomach, coming, as she expresses it, from the left side; the stitches are worst when making a mis-step.

" But if strong doses are renewed each day, and continued during a long time, besides the stomach pains, of which we have spoken, there manifests itself a species of *fever* exactly indicated by M. Bretonneau, *and which affects an intermittent type*, when the cinchona is given in an intermittent manner. *This fever is a species of vicious circle, in which very often inexperienced physicians turn, who are ignorant of the action of cinchona; they redouble the doses of the medicine, and throw the patient into a state which may be very serious."*

* W. T. Gardener, M.D., The Lancet, Nov. 17th, 1877.

"2. When lying down she feels quite well; she has then no pain anywhere, neither in the side nor in the pit of the stomach.

"3. She cannot sleep after three o'clock in the morning.

"4. She relishes her food, but after having eaten something she feels an inclination to vomit.

"5. When this inclination to vomit comes on, the water accumulates in her mouth and runs out of it as in waterbrash.

"6. After every meal she has several empty risings.

"7. She is of a vehement temper, disposed to be angry. When the pain is violent she is covered with sweat. Her menses are regular, and had ceased a fortnight ago.

"Bryonia deserves a preference over every other remedy in this case. As the woman was very robust, and as the forces of disease had affected her organism so painfully that she was not able to continue her work, and as, moreover, her vital powers were impaired, I gave her a full drop of the tincture of bryonia, with directions to see me again in forty-eight hours. I told my friend E——, who was present, that the woman's health ought to be restored after this period, which he doubted, not being yet fully converted to the new doctrine. In two days he returned to know the result, but the woman did not come. My friend, being impatient and determined to know what effect the medicine had produced, travelled to the village where the woman resided, to inform himself. He found the woman, and inquired of her why she had not returned?

4

But she replied, 'What should I do at the doctor's? Next day I was quite well and able to go about my washing, and ever since I have been as well as I am now. A thousand thanks to the doctor, but folks like me have no time to spare of their work; I had not earned a cent for three weeks past.' " *

This use of strong tinctures may be called the practice of his mature manhood, so unlike the whimsical speculations of his old age, when his mind could not brook the slightest opposition, nor admit of any independent investigation by any one of his followers, from whom he exacted a blind submission, which his early disciples most freely gave.

When cholera invaded Europe in 1831, Hahnemann prescribed camphor, *in large doses*, frequently repeated : at the time, too, when he was full of his idea of infinitesimal doses, which he recognized were not potent enough to grapple with that terrible disease. Refusing to extend his own experience of that disease to others nearly as deadly, he insisted upon ignoring the facts of experience to promulgate the whimsical notion of dynamization, begotten not of careful experiment, but of fanciful dogmatism, which denounced in harsh terms all who differed from him.

Truth† is greater than Hahnemann, and of late

---

* From the preface to the second volume of Hahnemann's Materia Medica Pura, Hempel's translation. Published by Radde, New York, and Ballière, London, 1846.

† " Some people suppose that a physician, professing belief in homœopathic law, is obliged to limit his practice strictly to the application of that law. He is not to administer a purgative,

years his speculations about "psora" and "infinitesimal doses" have been tacitly given up by all the most skilful and intelligent of his followers.

Following up Haller's idea of the necessity of the knowledge of the effects of medicines upon the healthy human body before applying them to the cure of disease, Hahnemann first sought for the law of cure, irrespective of any theory of disease. At a later period he fell into the old mistake which he so eloquently denounced in others. His own theory of psora was just as baseless as any of the many theories which he helped to overthrow.

Twenty-seven years ago I saw that the essential truth of Hahnemann's law was totally independent of his speculations about dynamization. Adopting with

-----

or to give an opiate, or to prescribe quinine, or to recommend a mineral water, under any circumstances, without in some way incurring the suspicion of sailing under false colors, of having deserted his creed and betrayed his principles. To those who cannot rise above the mere partisan spirit of cliques and schools, this may seem to be a righteous judgment. The man, however, who is loyal only to nature and to truth, regards such restrictions as sheer impertinence, and claims everything which *cures*, be the process explainable or not, as inalienably his own. He is astonished at the blindness and bigotry of the old school, who permit the grandest treasures of the curative art to lie unrecognized before them. He sets them a nobler example. He cultivates assiduously his own special field of science, but if he finds any residuum of truth or usefulness in allopathy, or any other system, he asks no man's permission to use it; but, acknowledging its source, appropriates it by divine right as the legitimate property of every healer of the sick."—Wm. H. Holcombe: Address before the Hahnemann Medical Society of Cincinnati, 1875.

great delight the law of "similia similibus curantur" as the chief, though not the only, foundation for therapeutics, I learnt for myself that Hahnemann's "sober" teaching, the use of the pure, undiluted tinctures, was a far better guide to heal the sick than Hahnemann "drunk" with mysticism, calling for the exclusive use of infinitesimal doses. The latter I gradually cast aside *in toto*, as untrustworthy and unjust to the sick, whose diseases too often remained stationary under treatment by globules, but were most effectually and quickly cured by tangible doses of the same medicines which failed to cure when given in infinitesimal doses.

Thus we see for the many centuries—from Hippocrates to Hahnemann—theories of treatment, all turning on theories of the nature of disease, or of the supposed nature or effects of medicines. Hence the uncertainty, because of the treacherous foundation upon man's thoughts and opinions, not upon facts.

The latter part of the eighteenth century was one of the darkest periods in the history of medicine. Large quantities of various drugs were mixed together, till the doctor's prescription became a source of hopeless confusion, obscuring all therapeutic science, and reducing the practice of medicine to a rough-and-ready art of crude drugging, to the neglect of physiological knowledge and hygiene.

At that period of imperfect light, when medicine was like a ship tossing on the ocean without a compass, the far-seeing eye of genius enabled Hahnemann to bring in an idea of infinite usefulness, which has spread over the entire region of medical practice, giving the

keynote to every great improvement in therapeutics
from his day to the present. Insensibly the practice
of physicians of all countries has been modified and
improved by the sharp, exclusive* teaching of Hahnemann.

Apart from all the mistakes, prejudices, and later
theories of the illustrious Hahnemann, the truth cannot be shaken that, in many cases, although not in all,
there is a relationship of similarity between the physiological action of the remedial agent and its essential
curative action. Interpretations (theories) may vary
and fall to the ground, the facts cannot perish, and
remain the surest guide to successful treatment, to
ignore which is destructive of success.

Dr. James Ross, in the *Practitioner* for October,
1870, describes the theory of "similia similibus" as
"my theory," omitting to add that "my theory" is
nearly word for word that of Samuel Hahnemann.†
Laws of therapeutics are built upon no man's theory,
but upon the sure foundation of facts, not needing
Hahnemann's theory, much less that of Dr. James
Ross, both of which may fall to the ground; yet the

---

* Hume's argument that "the intolerance of Christianity by
which it refused alliance with other religions, and insisted in
reigning alone or not at all, facilitated its reception," applies
with singular accuracy to the introduction and spread of homœopathy.

† Dr. Ringer, in his recent work on therapeutics, recom-
mends mercury in mumps, tonsillitis, and dysentery: and this is
only what might be anticipated if my theory is the correct one.
—Practitioner, Oct. 1870, "On the Action of Mercury," by
James Ross, M.D.

truth stands, that the action of medicinal agents in disease follows the relationship of similarity in most cases.

The time has come to dispense with hypothesis and theory. In medicine, the ultimate appeal must be to facts, which true science discovers, arranges, combines, and interprets. It is precious work to clear away the gross darkness of mock science, even when hid under an appearance of learning.

The need in the study of "materia medica pura" is to discover accurately the individual action of each remedial agent, to exclude all doubtful matter, so as to bring into clearer light the special characteristic of each, wherein its curative sphere lies. Also to find out the influences that oppose the direct or curative action, in order to remove or obviate their opposing influences.

The scientific or complete teaching of therapeutics should begin at the accurate knowledge of the effects of medicinal agents upon the healthy human body. The physiological action then becomes the key to accurate application of therapeutic agents in disease, the exact signs, symptoms, and causes of which being investigated, the student of medicine would learn a double diagnosis—that of the disease and of the medicinal agent most similar or most contrary to it. Thus accuracy of therapeutics would go *pari passu* with accuracy of medical knowledge, and "faith in medicine" become general. Exact knowledge is the only true remedy for heterodoxy. A large field is still left for the empirical skill of the doctor: indeed, a fruitful field to the diligent worker. The more fruitful the more he is experienced in the application of the great laws of therapeutics.

In the eighteenth century Cullen taught that the living body consists of a number of organs, each of which possesses powers of a specific nature, and that when irregularity occurs in the actions of the whole machine, either from internal or external causes, if it be not in an excessive degree, the self-regulating principle is sufficient to control the operation of the morbid cause, and to restore the system to its healthy condition.

This regulating principle, the "vis medicatrix naturae," differs essentially from the "Archæus" of Van Helmont, or the "Anima" of Stahl, inasmuch as it was supposed not to be anything superadded to the body, but one of the powers or properties necessary to its constitution as a living system. What may be called the Cullenian school of medicine comprehends a large portion of the most distinguished British physicians during the latter part of the eighteenth century. The rational empiricism, as it has been termed, which he so firmly established, superseded, in this country at least, the opposite extreme of speculation and hypothesis.

The early part of the nineteenth century is a most distinctive epoch in the history of therapeutics. The teaching of Brown cast a fresh light upon the practice of medicine. He attempted to explain all the phenomena of life and disease by a specific hypothesis of his own. Originally destined for the church, Brown never devoted himself to the elementary studies of medicine, but possessing natural genius, he set himself to the task of opposing the doctrines of Cullen. He assumed that the living body possesses a specific property, or power, termed " excitability ; " that everything which affects the living body acts upon this power as an excitant or stimulant. He assumed that the effect of this in its ordinary state is to produce the healthy condition of the functions : when excessive to cause exhaustion or direct debility ; when defective to produce indirect debility. He assumed that all morbid action depends upon one or other of these states of direct or indirect debility.

Accordingly he arranged diseases in two great classes of sthenic and asthenic, and directed treatment only to the general means for increasing or diminishing the excitement, without any regard to specific symptoms ; the only consideration he recognized being that of degree, the only measure that of quality. Brown, in the preface to his *Elements of Medicine*, relates how he wasted twenty years of his life in "learning, teaching, and diligently scrutinizing every part of medicine." That in his thirty-sixth year he had his first fit of gout. "For many years before he had lived well." It happened, however, that a few months before the attack of gout he had adopted a diet more sparing than usual. After the first attack " the disease did not return till six years later, and only then in consequence of unusual low living for several months."

The disease, according to the old theory, depended

upon plethora and excessive vigor; vegetable aliment was enjoined, wine was forbidden.

An entire year was passed in a strict adherence to this regimen. In that space of time he experienced no less than six fits of gout, and the whole year—except fourteen days—was divided between limping and excruciating pain.

If excess of vigor was the cause of the disease, according to the general theory, it became to him a subject of inquiry how such distressing symptoms were to be explained: why the disease had not made its first appearance twelve or fifteen years before, at a time when there was in reality more blood and vigor in the system, and why it only came on after a considerable reduction of his diet—why so great an interval, during which he had returned to his usual full diet, had intervened between the first fit and these recent ones? *

Brown paid but little attention to "diagnosis." His description of disease is very meagre and imperfect. His doctrine and practice were attractive to many by their plausibility. Dividing all diseases into two classes of sthenic and asthenic, his treatment was equally simple. Stimuli of different kinds for the asthenic; bleeding, low diet, and purging for the sthenic. The list of sthenic diseases is by far the smaller of the two in his classification.

The *Brunonian* system obtained many adherents

---

* Dr. Brown's Works. Edited by his son, 1804.

in this country. In Italy for some time it enjoyed considerable popularity.

Brown struck the keynote in the supporting system of medical practice. The fire of Brown's enthusiasm fell upon Graves, who, going round the wards of the Meath Hospital, once said to his class, " If anything is to be written on my tombstone, let it be: 'This man fed fevers.'" When the practice of most physicians in Europe was that of starving disease into subjection— mistaking the true significance of delirium, as if indicative of inflammation or congestion, to be treated by leeches and blisters to the head, with low diet—Graves taught that good food and the moderate use of alcohol cured many bad cases that the opposite system of treatment killed. His practice and teaching had a wonderful effect for good at the time when the genius and fire of Broussais was all-powerful for evil in Europe.*

The therapeutical teaching of Broussais† was the

---

* The early annals of the nineteenth century record a brilliant list of Frenchmen illustrious in physiology and pathology —Cuvier, Bichat, Majendie, Pinel, Andral, Louis. Germany at the same time produced physiologists and anatomists of great ability—Meckel, Wrisberg, Reil, Sprengel, etc. But while the labors of these distinguished men did great things for anatomy, physiology, and pathology, the treatment of disease received little or no help.

† Dr. J. Henry Bennett, coming fresh in 1846 from the Pathological School of Paris, where the destructive doctrines of Broussais still reigned, brought over to England the doctrine that most if not all diseases of the uterus were inflammatory and "ulcerative." Taken by surprise at the boldness and novelty of such one-sided views, the profession in England passively accepted a doctrine to which the opposition of weak

most violent reaction from Brown's doctrine. Of all the men of genius who ever practiced medicine, Broussais proved the most mischievous to humanity. In all diseases he saw inflammation of one sort or another, to be treated by low diet, leeching, and mild purgatives. Alas! "By your fruits ye shall know them." Soon the disciples of Broussais were recognized by the disastrous failure of their practice. In his own country it was reserved for Trousseau to lead the reaction against the starvation and lowering of Broussais. It was the teaching of Graves which gave the impetus to Trousseau, who looked upon the illustrious Irishman as his model. To those who knew what French medical and dietetic treatment was in Paris and its hospitals thirty years ago, the change seems like a transformation. When the murderous fire of the half drunken soldiers of the unhappy Louis Napoleon, in the *coup d'etat* of 1851, filled all the hospitals of Paris with wounded citizens, shot down at their doors and windows, the English visitors at the Paris hospitals were surprised to see meat, soup, and wine freely prescribed, and watched with interest the marvellous recoveries accomplished through the resources of "*restorative* surgery."

Dr. Hughes Bennett followed close upon Graves. His observation of the use of cod-liver oil in the hospitals in Germany, led him to recommend its use in

---

men like Dr. Robert Lee gave fresh but short-lived impetus. Left without active opposition during the past ten years, Dr. J. H. Bennett's "ulceration of the womb" doctrine has died a natural death.

pulmonary consumption. Dr. C. J. B. Williams quickly adopted the recommendation, and popularized it. Of all the discoveries of the present century, that has proved the greatest boon to suffering humanity. It helped to introduce the true idea of nutritive food into the treatment of disease. The well-merited fame of Dr. Hughes Bennett lies also in his total demolition* of that old fiction, "the change of type of disease," so long and so foolishly battled for by Dr. Alison and others, when the medical world was shocked by the bold and candid avowal of Sir John Forbes in 1845.†

It is of vital consequence to the true progress of medical science, that the rising generation of young doctors should not forget what medical practice was forty years ago in England. It is an instructive lesson to run the eye over the early editions of Sir Thomas Watson's *Principles and Practice of Medicine*, and to see what a prominent and constantly recurring place is occupied by such exploded things as bleeding, leeching, blistering, and mercury, till Dr. Hughes Bennett cut the foundation from under such scientific murder, and showed that pneumonia, a most deadly disease under the old *régime*, was curable by

---

* Not by declamation nor by setting opinion against opinion, but by the inexorable logic of facts was the victory won. In the annals of medicine, there is no story so telling, because true, as the records of Dr. Hughes Bennett's treatment of acute diseases in the Infirmary of Edinburgh.

† British and Foreign Review, No. 41: "Homœopathy, Allopathy, and Young Physic."

very simple means—careful dieting, perfect rest, and mild diuretics.

Dr. Todd proved himself an apt disciple of Graves, and in England helped to overthrow the expiring but tenacious energy of strong drugging and weak feeding in medical practice. Dr. Todd's teaching at King's College had the best influence upon therapeutics. Although endeavoring to put the use of alcoholic fluids upon a true scientific basis, he got the credit of prescribing such in excessive doses,* and the want of success in his hospital results caused a partial reaction after his death.

After Dr. Todd in England, followed the vigorous blows of Dr. King Chambers, in his lectures upon the " Renewal of Life." Where Todd was inclined to push the use of alcohol at times to an unsafe point, Dr. King Chambers fell into the same mistake as regards overfeeding in acute diseases, in typhoid fever especially.

At Bartholomew's, Skey helped the progress of sus-

---

* The pupils of Dr. Todd have accomplished what their illustrious master endeavored to do : to place the administration of alcohol upon a scientific basis. Practical medicine owes a debt of gratitude to Dr. Anstie and Dr. Dupré, for their accurate and most reliable experiments upon the use of alcoholic fluids. No unprejudiced mind can now doubt that the action of alcohol in moderate doses is that of food to be oxidized in the human body, and leads to the production of force. Their experiments have demonstrated to a certainty that only a minute portion passes out of the economy unchanged, when the quantity taken is in moderate doses, not exceeding two ounces of absolute alcohol in twenty-four hours.

taining the vital force in disease, but in private practice he got a very bad name for the indiscriminate
recommendation of alcoholic stimulants.   Of one of
his contemporaries given to the same indiscriminate
use of wine, it was said, "he made more drunkards
than any man living," a sad and most solemn reproach ;
a humiliating yet true warning to the rising generation
of medical practitioners.   With few exceptions, the
medical profession in Great Britain has adopted the
supporting system, so much so that at the present time
it requires courage and sound judgment not to oppress
the sick man's stomach with too much food, and not
to *narcotize* the brain with too large doses of wine or
brandy.   It is often most difficult to prevent anxious
friends and nurses overdoing "support."   A wise physician, practicing in Bristol, relates that he was for
many days giving the utmost amount of nourishment
and stimulant to a severe case of acute disease.   When
the nurses and friends thought the patient dying, he
was summoned at two o clock in the morning.   She
lay unconscious in a stupor, breathing hurriedly, pulse
fluttering, and neck and face livid.   On inquiry, he
found that the full quantity of nourishment and stimulant had been regularly given since his last visit, at
10 P.M.   By a sudden thought, he asked for ice.   He
stood by the bedside of one to all appearance dying,
and for twelve hours gave nothing but ice-water, and
she most unexpectedly recovered.

From England and France an influence for good has
very slowly spread into Italy, where the last stronghold
of the bleeding and starvation system of treatment held

out long after it had been struck down in the greater part of the civilized world. It was not till the death of Cavour that the inert public opinion of Italy was roused to recognize the horrors of the old orthodox destructive medicine, with its rich ornamentation of bleeding, leeching, starving, tartar emetic, and laxatives. Italy can now show many skilful physicians and surgeons who have exchanged bleeding, leeches, and tartar emetic for good food, red wine, and skilful medication.

A new era in the elucidation of the knowledge of the nervous system was inaugurated by Dr. Brown-Séquard, one of the most original of all investigators in the domain of physiology and therapeutics. His discovery of the true functions of the ganglionic centres and of the vaso-motor nerves comes next in its marvellous results to Harvey's discovery of the circulation of the blood. The physician, occupied in the daily routine of medical practice, looks on and wonders at the rich results of such a life of labor in the fields of science.

Brown-Séquard's researches have been admirably followed up by Drs. Frazer, Crum-Brown, Brunton, and Ringer, furnishing us with most minute and accurate details, yet, alas! afraid to teach the laws or fundamental principles which underlie the science of therapeutics.

When Brown-Séquard, the distinguished man of science, settled down to practice medicine in Cavendish Square and at the National Hospital for the Paralyzed and Epileptic, he quickly showed that the ac-

curacy of the man of science was not incompatible with
the skilful practice of medicine, and that the most
minute and delicate experiments upon animals were
to throw a flood of light upon the medicinal treatment
of the diseases of man.   Many epileptic and many paralyzed patients have had cause to bless the labors of
the man who for so many years patiently experimented
upon guinea pigs and rabbits in the causation of epilepsy and paralysis.

It is pleasant to know that the use of chloroform
aided Brown-Séquard by annulling pain in the animals on which he experimented.   His discoveries of
the exact, indeed the ultimate, action of belladonna,
ergot, strychnia, and bromide of potassium would alone
entitle him to the gratitude of all physicians.   Whilst
demonstrating the portion of the nervous system upon
which each of those medicines acts, he seems to conceive
of no relationship of that action in health to its use in
disease, but the Galenical notion of " contraria contrariis," and hence the large doses, bordering upon semi-
poisonous, which he advises.

With the name of Laennec is connected the first and
most important of all discoveries of the nineteenth century in the improvement of diagnosis of the diseases of
the heart, lungs, and bloodvessels—the stethoscope ;
the first of the physical aids to diagnosis, the precursor
of many others, the ophthalmoscope, laryngoscope,
sphygmograph, and the clinical thermometer.

" Every true work of the man of science is a fruitful one, and often leads to fresh discoveries."   When
the greatest of living physical philosophers, Helmholtz,

discovered the ophthalmoscope, and handed it over to the oculist for use, few even of the latter conceived what a boon to suffering humanity, what a help in the diagnosis and treatment, this wonderful instrument would prove. All the knowledge of the eye and its diseases which the previous twenty centuries had accumulated, sinks into insignificance when compared with the discoveries of the past twenty years. The name of Von Graafe, and the cure of glaucoma by iridectomy, are intimately associated with the use of the ophthalmoscope.

The skill of this man of genius (Von Graafe) led to the discovery of the successful results of iridectomy in the treatment of glaucoma, but it bids fair to be brought into disrepute from the indiscriminate use made of it. Ophthalmic surgeons perform it for many diseases of the eye other than glaucoma. In the latter its effects are little short of marvellous, but in many other cases more harm than good seems to result from the operation.

The laryngoscope, although the discovery of a German (Zermach), has derived its best application in disease from the energy and skill of an English physician —Dr. Morell Mackenzie—who has done much to exhibit its great power in the treatment of diseases of the throat and larynx.

The clinical use of the thermometer in disease, so admirably worked out by Wunderlich, has much increased the precision of diagnosis in many diseases, especially in typhoid fever and acute rheumatism. It has done still more for prognosis, and has prepared the way for a more accurate science of hydropathy.

The knowledge that high temperature indicated waste and exhaustion of the muscular tissues of the body and of the heart, naturally suggested the use of cold baths to reduce the temperature.*

The modern American Eclectic school has introduced into medical practice many most valuable medicines, especially podophyllin, leptandrin, gelsemin, and hydrastis; but like most attempts at eclecticism, losing all anchorage of "first principles" of therapeutics, it has degenerated into the most indiscriminate drugging with enormous doses of the most nauseous medicines mixed up together in inextricable confusion.

The true physician should, like Lord Bacon, aim at the acquisition of all knowledge, and when knowledge comes, wisdom should not linger. He must not degenerate into eclecticism, which is a mere collection of details without law and without any true basis on which to develop. The recollection of a multitude of individual cures can be of but uncertain use till codified by laws, thenceforth to help the creation of science in place of perishing with the man and his use of them.

Claude Bernard's demonstration of the effects of section of the sympathetic nerve in the neck, marks an era in physiology most instructive to the physician. Here for the first time the actual phenomena of inflammation became practically visible; no longer the opinion of a man, but observed fact. Destroy, or para-

---

* Lancet.

lyze, or weaken the power of the vaso-motor nerves, or
of their ganglionic centres, and the bloodvessels are
deprived of the nervous force by which their muscular
fibres are ruled. Hence undue relaxation of their
coats, and what was for so many centuries called "inflammation" ensues. Distended bloodvessels, swollen
structures, increased heat, and increased secretion fill
up the picture of the old writers, with whom swelling,
redness, heat, constituted the essentials of inflammation.

In the beginning of the present century the word
inflammation hung like a dark cloud over the horizon
of therapeutics; invariably associated with danger and
with the need for "antiphlogistic" treatment, sugges-
tive of bleeding, leeching, blistering, low diet—agents
that keep up a state of terror in the doctor's mind as
well as in that of the patient. Ignorant of the processes
at work in the disturbed economy, it was difficult for
the doctor* to feel at ease, especially when finding the
uselessness of his vigorous means of destruction.

The "dyscrasia" doctrines of the Vienna school
tended to fix upon the blood and the fluids as the source
of disease. To its credit it begat caution in the use of
lowering means, and courage in the doctors. Courage
to stand by and watch the course of disease, undisturbed
by "antiphlogistic treatment."

The dyscrasia doctrine of the Vienna school was

---

* When scarcely any one in this country dared to allow an
acute disease to run its course without the interference of powerfully perturbing medicines.—Practitioner, iv, 228.

vague and unsatisfactory. In the present day a true regard is paid to the state of the blood and of its constituents, the character of the albumen, and the proportion and condition of its inorganic salts. This again leads back to a more exact examination of the food and the condition of the digestive and assimilative organs. In this direction the key to the "degenerations" of the structures must be sought. Excess of food may prove a more fertile source of degeneration than the opposite. If the albumen be thick, over rich, it may afford a worse pabulum to the tissues than a lighter quality derived from *poorer* food.

The genius of Virchow pushed aside the dyscrasia doctrine, and fixed attention too exclusively on the tissues of the body, finding the growth of cells sufficient to explain all the phenomena of inflammation and nutrition.

The discovery by Cohnheim, in 1867, of the passage of white blood-corpuscles through the unruptured walls of the capillaries, the change of these white corpuscles into pus-cells, demonstrated the necessity of regarding the state of the fluids as well as of the tissues.

The most important result of Cohnheim's demonstration upon therapeutics is the use of quinine by Dr. Binns, of Bonn, to arrest this proliferation of white corpuscles, and their transformation into pus-cells.

Truth is an ungrudging helper, gives freely, abundantly, to all who enter her portals with a simple and teachable spirit. The best scholars in that school are the first to claim nothing for themselves, but modestly to acknowledge the source of their gathering. Science has its nobles as well as its commoners.

In the history of medicine for twenty-three centuries, *i.e.*, from the age of Hippocrates to the eighteenth century, we see physicians in every age founding their treatment on their *opinions* as to the nature of disease, not on facts : hence the uncertainty and vagueness of the science and art of healing. One age struggling to cast down the theory of disease and system of treatment of the previous age.

Hippocrates, with all the grand instincts of genius, photographing, as it were, in words the natural history of disease, yet founding his system of treatment upon his *opinion* of the nature of disease. The various sects springing up after his decease doing in their way just what Hippocrates did. Therapeutics continue confused and hazy till Galen steps in with great force of character to teach the distinct and positive dogma of "contraria contrariis curantur." With this sharply-defined principle, unfortunately, opinions as to the nature of disease, and the qualities of medicines, displaced accurate observation of facts.

Galen's doctrines differed little from Hippocrates's except in their sharply-defined character and their fierceness.

Therapeusis, all through the many centuries of the decline and fall of the Roman Empire, is but the *echo* of Galen ; re-echoed all through the Middle Ages, and right on to the eighteenth century, when Haller led physicians back to the study of nature—physiology— as the only true basis of the science of medicine.

In all this important work the present century has advanced with rapid strides. Preventive medicine has done much to investigate the cause, especially of epidemic diseases. Armed with this knowledge of the cause, it quickly meets the invader, isolates and roots it out before it has time to spread. In this way the silent work of saving thousands of precious lives goes on from day to day.

Preventive medicine has found its truest disciples in England. The investigation of the cause of disease has borne rich and abundant fruit. The example of the late Dr. Snow's life is a good proof that prosperity in the pursuit of medical practice need not interfere with scientific investigation. Fully and profitably occupied in the very narrow specialty of chloroform administration, he had genius to search out the cause of cholera, and the industry to follow it up to actual demonstration in the drinking-water from the memorable pump near Golden Square, close to the spot where lay the dead bodies of thousands who died in the Great Plague.

CHAPTER II.

PHYSIOLOGY.

In the earliest stage of society there are many arts, but no sciences. A little later science begins to appear, and every subsequent step is marked by an increased desire to bring art under the dominion of science.*

We only reach the province of science when we ascend beyond the description of mere phenomena to their laws, the comprehensive order or combinations of order which the phenomena obey.†

In its simplest sense law is but the observed order of facts, not requiring that the cause of the same should be known. Mathematicians and astronomers accustomed to deal with the highest, i.e., the most fixed order of facts, are satisfied to accept the law of gravitation, although the cause of that law has not yet been discovered.

"Astronomy has been a brilliant example for the development of the other branches of science. In its case, by the theory of gravitation, a vast and complex mass of facts were first embraced in a single principle of great simplicity, and such a reconciliation of theory and fact established as has never been accomplished in

---

* Buckle, Fraser's Magazine, April, 1858.
† Comte, Edinburgh Review, April, 1868.

any other department of science, neither before or since."*

" The forces which determine chemical combination all work under rules as sharp and definite as the force of gravitation ; so do the forces which operate in light and heat, and sound, in magnetism and electricity."

Before Dalton's grand discovery† of the atomic theory, chemistry was a mere empirical art, full of hypotheses and uncertain opinions, exactly in the same position which therapeutics occupies in the present day. When the genius of Dalton discovered that each chemical element united to others in definite proportions, then indeed the atomic theory placed chemistry in the front rank of the exact sciences.

In the short time (eighty years) since Dalton discovered the law of atomic weight or proportions, chem-

---

* Helmholtz, Popular Lectures on Scientific Subjects, p. 26.

† The three grand laws of constant proportions, multiple proportions, and reciprocal proportions were traced out by Richter, Berzelius, and others before Dalton's time.

But to him belongs the credit of having clearly stated and explained these three laws. He suggested that " matter was not infinitely divisible, but was composed of minute particles or atoms having an invariable character."

His investigations extended over the years 1804–8.

" Upon this hypothesis (Dalton's atomic theory) the ultimate particles of each element are considered to be uniform in size and in weight for that element, and, moreover, to be incapable of further subdivision. When bodies unite chemically, as the particles of the same element have all the same size and relative weight, the proportions in which they combine must be definite; and further, if they unite in several different proportions, those proportions must be simply related to each other."
—Miller's Chemical Physics, pp. 15–16.

istry has made more progress than it had previously during thousands of years.

The discovery of the law of the development of all parts of the flower from leaves in different stages of development, introduced the most wonderful unity and simplicity into the science of botany. " The elementary floret," we are told (Lewes's *Life of Goethe*, vol. ii, p. 145), " expands into a leaf upon the stem, contracts to make the calyx, expands again to make the petal, to contract once more into sexual organs, and expand for the last time into fruit."*

Goethe gave the first impulse to the researches of comparative anatomy into the analogy of corresponding organs in different animals, and to the parallel theory of the metamorphosis of leaves in the vegetable kingdom ; and thus, in fact, really pointed out the direction which the science has followed ever since.†

The same lesson of law which astronomy, chemistry, and botany teach, is exemplified by physiology, which deals with more complex phenomena than chemistry, inasmuch as the simplest living being presents conditions more complicated and more variable than any merely chemical phenomena. Man is the highest product of nature, the highest form of nature's most complex organization.‡ The development, growth,

---

* " Plants and animals present a striking difference, in the fact that plants can manufacture fresh protoplasm out of mineral compounds ; whereas animals are obliged to procure it ready-made, and hence in the long run depend upon plants."—Huxley, Fortnightly Review, February, 1869.

† Helmholtz, Popular Lectures on Scientific Subjects, p. 20.

‡ " That we might be a kind of first fruits of his creatures."

functions, reproduction, and decay of a living organism, cause us to stand still and wonder at the Infinite Wisdom that set such marvellous processes into action, and keeps them going through their appointed existence.

In the first development of human life, we see the embryo as a single cell, the ovum set free from the ovary; passing along the Fallopian tube, it reaches its receptacle, the uterus, where it finds everything favorable for its life: warmth, moisture, rest.   Yet it abides alone, it dies, unless it meets its correlative cell, the spermatozoon, analogous to itself, yet different.

After the fertilizing action of the spermatozoon, the impregnated ovum finds in the uterus everything suitable for its development and growth.   Abundant bloodvessels, the contents of which the thin, delicate structures of the placenta allow to pass into those of the ovum.   This receives its nourishment from the blood, a complex fluid containing upwards of twenty different ingredients, selecting with unfailing accuracy only what is akin to its own structures, appropriating those and refusing all others ;* the skin, cellular tissue, glands, converting and aggregating to themselves the fibrin and albumen, the rudimentary skeleton absorbing the earthy salts.

We find the law of development to be like appropriating like.

---

* " The development of organs withdraws from the blood some element of nutrition, which if retained in it would be positively injurious, like a retained excretion."—Sir J. Paget's Hunterian Lectures.

In growth we can trace the young child after birth living upon the food provided for it—milk—the only food which contains all the principles essential to life and growth. The infant structures grow by selecting with unerring accuracy from the blood, the materials akin to their own composition.* Invariably, insensibly, and unerringly, each tissue selects the material akin to itself, and rejects all else, for use to some other organ that needs it. Year by year, up to mature age, the bones absorb more earthy salts, and the soft cartilaginous structures become harder and stronger, able to sustain the weight of the body; the muscles become firmer and more active, the skin more tense and thick, the convolutions of the brain deeper and larger as the mental faculties develop and are exercised. Every organ and structure obeys the physiological law that moderate use strengthens and expands an organ, if the conditions of supply are natural. As years go on to adult life, we see the greater activity of life-processes demands a more abundant supply of nourishment. Increased activity of assimilation makes up for increased work of organs and more rapid decay of tissues.

---

* Equally wonderful as is the process of growth in the animal kingdom is it in the vegetable. " In any rocky pool when the tide is out, we may find the graceful plants which we call sea weeds, sipping from the mingled waters their daily fractional dose of iodine. Housed sea-snails sucking from it carbonate of lime for their shells, restless fishes extracting from it phosphate of lime to strengthen their bones, and lazy-like sponges, dipping successfully into it for silica, to distend the mouths of their filters."—Dr. George Wilson.

When the activity of life wanes, the power of absorption and assimilation lessens.

The organs whose vital force is weakest, first feel the change. The hair becomes white, the skin loses its activity, shrivels, the arcus senilis shows the organic or nutritive force yielding, and the inorganic force—the chemical—asserting its power over the vital force, indicating that the same process is probably at work in the valves of the heart and in the coats of the arteries.

The chemical force seems to block up the vessels and strangle the organic force, the feebleness of which allows the prop to be taken from under the animal life, and thus death comes, when natural, through the organ by whose inherent weakness the working power first fails.

What a marvellous idea of the wisdom and power of God, that this capacity for selection pervades every tissue and every organ of the living body, and that for centuries—aye, for scores of centuries—an unchanging law has watched over every organ and function. Men's and women's bodies were just the same as to organs, development, structure then as now.

"*If, then, we study the earliest indisputable specimens of fossil-men, we invariably find a man just such as men are now. The old Troglodytes, the dwellers in pile-villages and others, prove to be an exceedingly respectable society. If we take the sum of all the known fossil-men and compare them with man as he now exists, we can positively assert that among living men there is a far greater number of relatively inferior individuals than among the fossils which are as yet known.*"—Professor Virchow, *Quarterly Review*, January, 1878.

The same laws of health and disease existed in the time of the ancient Assyrians, Greeks, and Romans, as obtain at the present hour in the denizens of our towns. The comparison of ancient sculpture and drawings seems to verify the belief that men and women were precisely the same thousands of years ago, not the least stronger or more healthy, not more free from disease than the present generation. In ancient pictures and sculptures there is the same evidence of the scrofulous constitution which is so easily recognized and so often met with at the present day. The very diseases which Hippocrates describes are identically the same as those to which the human body is now liable. The same causes and influences were then at work in the production of those diseases as are now recognized; the same muscles, the same joints, the same brains, eyes, ears, and senses. From century to century the laws* of growth and assimilation remain, ever unerring and unchangeable.

"Nature does not allow us for a moment to doubt that we have to do with a rigid chain of cause and effect. Therefore to us, as her students, goes forth the mandate to labor on till we have discovered unvarying laws." †

A monster has become a term synonymous with a

---

* " Measurement of ancient armor and clothes show that we are bigger, measurements of athletic feats show that we are stronger than our ancestors."—Quarterly Review.

† Helmholtz, Popular Lectures, p. 23.

rare occurrence. Nature is so true to herself that the occasional aberration of law is regarded as a horrible thing out of due course; and yet physicians live in perpetual contact with those exquisite and unchanging facts and laws of physiology, but are content to grope and hit at random in their attempts to treat disease, not looking for principles of cure or definite laws in the selection of curative agents, satisfied, in fact, to make a good hit, if not to try again.*

The natural functions of the human body may be called work of organs. When we trace out the law of work or function we find each organ throwing off what is analogous to its own nature. The skin freely perspiring throws out of the body water, in which salts analogous to, or identical with, its own composition are dissolved. The liver and lungs exhale carbon as carbonic acid and bile. If one fails in its work, the other takes on itself extra work, or work of compensation.

The mucous membrane of the gastro-intestinal canal throws off particles of itself, epithelial scales, mixed with water and saline ingredients. Its work or function seems to be to shed its own surface and reproduce it again in a perpetual routine, day and night; if moderate, i. e., natural, just enough to lubricate the passages and carry impurities or secretions out of the body; if excessive, it becomes diarrhœa.

---

* A celebrated Italian physician, after forty years of medical practice, said, on his death-bed, "The doctor is like a man with a stiletto in a dark room with the patient and the disease, stabbing vigorously, but not knowing whether he strikes the disease or the patient."

"The work done by food in the body may be divided into the work of growth, the work of animal heat, mechanical work, and vital work." * In childhood and youth nutrition is most active to provide meterials for the growth of the various organs of the body, and in a less degree for work. In adult life the amount of food required for growth is much less, but more for the work of the organs. It is true that all work of organs is accompanied with destruction and metamorphosis of tissue, thus the food passes out of the body in the shape of work done.

---

* Professor Haughton on the " Relation of Food to Work:" The Lancet, p. 210, 1868.

CHAPTER III.

PATHOLOGY.

" But knowledge is not the sole object of man upon
earth.   Action alone gives a man a life worth living;
and therefore he must aim either at the practical application of his knowledge, or at the extension of the
limits of science itself."*

In the "Talmud" there is a saying, " Whosoever
does not increase in knowledge decreases." Physiology, the true foundation of all knowledge of disease,
bids fair to become one of the most exact of sciences.
Alas! that the superstructure, the treatment of disease,
should lag behind and be regarded, even by some of
its best disciples, as only an art, not possessing nor requiring exact laws.   To the mind of the physiologist
every process of the human body, its development,
assimilation, growth, reproduction, functions, secretions, decay, etc., obey in the most marvellous way the
action of definite laws; but when the physiologist
changes into the physician, forgetting the reign of law
in physiology, and not looking for definite laws of cure
in medicine, he rests satisfied with arbitrary rules and
opinions; hence comes the uncertainty in medical prac-

---

* Helmholtz, Popular Lectures on Scientific Subjects, p. 26.

tice and the want of success in the treatment of disease.

When acute disease affects a human body whose organs are all sound, nature, even in the worst cases, struggles towards recovery; but when one or more organs of the body are unsound, then the natural efforts to cure frequently struggle in vain, and at each stage of the struggle the tendency toward failure becomes the more evident. To take the simplest case, that of severe chill from exposure to cold. The functions of the skin being repressed, the natural force of the organism reacts vigorously upon the affected surface, free perspiration comes, and restoration to health follows. If the skin is dry and the health low, this result does not follow; but increased work of the kidney—the organ whose function is most akin to that of the skin—is set up, and a copious flow of dark urine relieves the system. If the kidneys are unable to respond in a sufficient degree, then nature calls out the curative action of that organ which is next in degree of affinity to the organ first affected, and free action of the liver and gastro-intestinal mucous membrane relieves the disease by natural diarrhœa. If the first and second in affinity cannot respond to the call, the diseased action becomes more profound, and falls upon the third and more remote function: then, especially if the heart is weak, pleurisy with effusion results. Unfortunately, the doctor seldom sees the patient till it is too late to cut short the disease. The physical signs too clearly indicate the progress towards effusion; the relief through the mucous membranes failing, the weight of the diseased action now falls upon the serous membranes. The effusion of pleurisy is often carried off naturally by the occurrence of diarrhœa or of free diuresis.

The organ which is quickest to respond to the strain of a diseased action upon another organ receives the curative impetus, and if active and healthy, saves the organism from further mischief; but if the energy of its nerve-force is low, or its vessels or tissues obstructed, it proves unequal to the vicarious action, and itself becomes diseased; as when the reaction of chill from the surface of the skin causes pneumonia, the effort of the lungs to right the system proving unequal, and their own structure suffering. The delicate cells of the lungs have to go through the process of consolidation, and subsequent absorption of the effused products of inflammation. Then the correlative organ, the liver, comes to the rescue, and excretes the carbon as a fluid, which the lungs are unable to do in a sufficient degree as a gas.

Congestion of the liver most easily relieves itself by increased action of the gastro-intestinal mucous membrane, to the structure of which the liver has the closest similarity. Failing this relief the effect of cure is thrown upon the lungs and skin. Nature calls out all the allied functions to help, each in its own degree of similarity or fitness. If one member suffer all the members suffer with it—that "the members should have the same care one for another."

Inaction of liver finds relief through free action of the lungs, promoted by brisk open-air exercise. An hour or two on horseback more than doubles the excretion of carbonic acid through the lungs—thus freeing the venous blood from the carbon which the liver is unequal to excrete.

Vascular obstruction (portal congestion) of the liver, finds a vent in bleeding piles, or else in hæmatemesis. Irritability of the biliary ducts provokes increased action of the same structures in the duodenum and ileum which relieves the liver. This would seem to be the true explanation of the action of mercury and of podophyllin in disease of the liver. The experiments of the Edinburgh Committee prove that mercury does not increase the flow of bile in dogs. The same probably obtains in the human subject also; but it is quite clear to any practical physician that mercury and podophyllin increase the secretion of the glands and mucous membrane of the small intestines. By the sympathy of action it generally provokes free secretion from the gall-bladder also.

In disease of the kidneys the first effort of nature to cure is through the skin. When free perspiration occurs early, and continues for some time, it is often sufficient to cure many cases of nephritis after scarlatina. Free action of the skin allows the tubuli uriniferi to rest from work, whilst the products of the kidney secretions are eliminated through the skin. An abundant supply of fluid—either pure water or milk—washes out the *débris* of the minute tubes, the albumen gradually disappears, and the urine becomes restored to its natural condition. The disease is cured without injury to the structure of the kidneys. This fortunate result seldom obtains, except in recent cases uncomplicated with degeneration.

When the skin is dry and inactive, so as to oppose her efforts, nature is driven to make use of the second in affinity, and selects the mucous membrane of the gastro-intestinal canal, setting up diarrhœa; but the relief through the second analogue is not so effectual as through the first, and the disease is not so effectually cured as when free diaphoresis carries off the dropsy.

When disease of kidney is not cured in the early stage, dropsy into the cellular tissue ensues, indicating that the diseased action is more intense, and still seeking relief through the skin, the organ most closely allied to the diseased one. It is a singular illustration of how nature works most frequently through the organ first in relationship of similarity to the organ diseased, that even in advanced stages of dropsy from kidney disease, it keeps chiefly to the cellular tissues to the last. From the lower extremities it spreads to the upper. In like manner œdema of the abdomen appears long before ascites or hydrothorax; œdema of the eyelids and face before effusion into the ventricles of the brain. An apparent exception to this occurs in advanced cases of granular degeneration, where the copious flow of urine, incidental to that form of kidney disease, prevents the coming on of œdema, yet towards the close of life effusion into the ventricles does occur, often without external dropsy.

Congestion of the brain often finds spontaneous relief in epistaxis, or in bleeding piles. The old practice of copious bleeding from the arm was wrong in principle, inasmuch as it was not seeking to relieve in the direction nature selects; so to speak, it was trying to relieve by a side stroke, not by a direct help. It was also most mischievous, as it paralyzed the vaso-motor nerves, and thus led to the extravasation of blood into the brain structure, which it was intended to arrest, but which in reality it precipitated.

To stand before nature and ask questions, we must accept the answers given, and act accordingly. A leech or two to the nostrils, in such cases, will do more good than the withdrawal of a quart of blood from the arm. Woe to the patient with congestion of brain, when medical science degenerates into expectancy, and when the doctor neglects true curative means till blood has been extravasated into the brain to damage its structure for the rest of life! What a solemn responsibility to the physician who, himself, might be the patient in such a predicament! Recovering after the solemn visit of the expectancy doctor, what a pang of agony that it was " recovering " with paralysis for the rest of life —a damaged brain, never again to work as of old!*

---

* At Pisa, in 1849, I visited an old English physician, a bed-ridden paralytic. " Let me give you one caution," said he. " I practiced for many years at Nice, and year after year I saw strong men struck down with paralysis and apoplexy, and I never warned such to keep away from Nice till I was struck down myself. Ever since it has been a cause of keen regret, aye, of bitter self-reproach. Let me beg you to warn middle-aged persons, if at all plethoric or excitable, that the climate of the Riviera—at least near the shore—is most disturbing to the brain."

CHAPTER IV.

THE NATURAL HISTORY OF DISEASE.

Facts, and the invariable laws which govern them, are the pursuit, and the only legitimate pursuit, of science.*

As we observe the work of nature in development, assimilation, growth, we see how invariable are the facts of physiology, how positive and clear the co-ordination of these facts; let us now watch how nature acts in disease, which is but a disturbance of the natural force of the body. Disease seldom is a special entity that finds entrance into the human body. In most cases it is but the natural functions of life disturbed—force more frequently lessened than increased.

In some cases disease is indeed a very positive entity from without—such as the poison of cholera, typhoid fever, or typhus. The origin and mode of entrance of such distinct disease-producer is well known to be dissolved in drinking-water, inhaled as sewer-gas, or absorbed by the lungs and skin. It is fashionable nowadays for every clever writer to explain that disease is not an "entity or substance," like "cats and dogs" in the words of Miss Nightingale. It would

---

* Comte, Edinburgh Review.

be a radical mistake to accept such doctrines in all cases. It would stay the search for the antidote to such diseases as cholera, typhus, typhoid fever, or scarlatina. It is quite possible yet that the skill of the chemical physiologist may discover some soluble disinfectant that, set free in the blood,—as chloral hydrate when decomposed by the alkaline salts of the blood,— may neutralize and stay the ravages of cholera and of typhoid fever. If the analogue to scarlatina could be discovered in some of the lower animals, inoculation therewith might prove as true a preventive of scarlatina as vaccination of small-pox.

Many, if not most, cases of acute diseases have a natural tendency to run a regular course, which frequently ends in recovery; the more so, the more the physician abstains from lowering or disturbing treatment, and the more naturally the strength of the patient is kept up by a full but not excessive amount of nutriment. Such cases seem to be cured by a simple subsidence or passing away of all the phenomena; yet with this natural tendency towards recovery in some cases, in others there is constant liability to death, or injury to vital organs, which needs all the watchful care and discerning judgment of the physician to know when the progress of the disease is deathwards, and what the interference of art can do to avert this tendency. It is true any treatment will cure simple diseases of an acute character, but it is equally true that a large proportion of the most intractable chronic diseases to which the human body is liable cannot be cured without direct medication that acts on the organ or

function diseased. How many cases of pericarditis
that end in adhesion, injuring the heart for life, would
be arrested in the early stage by a blister!

Art may prove a friend to help, or a foe to wound.
When the doctor gets out of the antagonistic attitude,
he soon finds that to act as a friend is to gain a helper.
Yet disease is seldom a natural process for the physician to stand idle and look on with folded hands, but
a disturbed natural process wanting a distinct knowledge of positive therapeutics to help at the right moment.

How often do we see the energetic practitioner, unable to find the key, trying, in vain, to open the casket
with smart blows of a hammer. On the other side
stands the mild disciple of modern expectant medicine
for months watching the casket, examining the lock,
but unable to find the key, till, to his horror, the
friends bring in a more dexterous operator. The cure
of the disease soon speaks for the perfect workman.
Like a jewel-case, which can be safely opened only by
one key, disease has often to be unlocked. A cure is
not accomplished till the special key is found.

In modern times, a class of physicians has arisen,
pluming themselves on their extra-scientific character,
who think it the highest attainment of medical art to
stand by and do nothing but "let Nature cure the disease." Many, very many, cases of acute, and thousands of cases of chronic, disease, however, will not
yield to expectant "treatment," even when the patient
is kept at rest, physiological and mechanical, carefully
preserved from all disturbing influences, well supplied

with nourishment, and drinking freely of mint-water to make him believe he is taking medicine. It is then that the gift of healing, which the true physician derives from the knowledge of principles or laws of cure, comes in to assist in extricating the patient from the tendency towards death or destruction of organs.

Expectant treatment, or mild medicine, has much to answer for at the bar of humanity. In December, 1869, I was summoned to Windsor, at midnight, to witness a sad illustration of *let alone* treatment. I found the patient, aged seventy, suffering from a severe attack of broncho-pneumonia, and was informed that for four days he had been under the treatment of the most celebrated of the London expectant treatment doctors. The only medicine given was spirit of mindererus. As he was getting daily worse, the patient's friends sent for Dr. Harper, who, alarmed by the dangerous predicament of the patient, telegraphed for me. Although a north wind was blowing, and the night frosty, I found the old man in a large, cold room, with a very small fire. He was semi-comatose from difficult and frequent respiration ; face purple ; feet œdematous and cold ; constantly coughing, and with great difficulty expectorating much frothy blood ; urine scanty and dark ; bowels confined for four days ; the left side of the chest was dull on percussion from base to apex ; respiratory murmur feeble, and crepitation general. By the aid of large fires, surrounded with wet sheets, the air of the room was warmed and softened. The sheets were removed from the bed, and each of the lower extremities

7

packed in dry hot flannel, then the body wrapped closely in blankets; large mustard poultices were applied along the spine and loins; yolk of egg beaten up with brandy was given freely to rouse the sinking heart; ten drops of tincture of squills was administered every quarter of an hour, from midnight till 5 A.M., when the oppression of breathing and stupor gradually lessened as the expectoration became free and the surface of the body warm and perspiring. At 8 A.M. all danger was over, and in twenty-four hours my friend Dr. Harper wrote: "I am glad to be able to report a *very* decided improvement: pulse 83, respirations 22. His cough has become easy, the breathing much relieved. His appearance is indeed marvellously changed for the better."

Hospital physicians, accustomed chiefly to recent cases of disease, mostly of subacute nature, find good feeding and nursing, plenty of fresh air, and perfect rest, do so much for their patients—often moved from homes devoid of any hygienic attribute to the large airy wards of the hospital—that they are apt to lose faith in medicine. To them it is much to abstain from the routine of evil drugging, the contrast of their results is so decidedly favorable in comparison with the bleeding, blistering, and generally lowering treatment of an age not quite gone by; but away from the hospital, amongst varied and perplexing chronic diseases, the fashion of "skepticism with regard to drugs" avails but little. There these "expectant medicine doctors" cut a poor figure, dealing in generalities of diet and nursing that avail but little to cure disease. In private practice, the physician finds it is not enough to advise a generous diet, with a good supply of wine, beer, or brandy ; good nursing and ventilation with a placebo of mint-water or lavander spirit.   The disease will not yield—the friends get impatient.   Accurate knowledge of principles of therapeutics is wanted in order to grapple with the disease, which the patient wants to be cured of as speedily as possible.   This neglect of therapeutics reacts upon the public and the medical profession ; upon the public in their dislike of the doctor and his physic. How clever it is thought to get the doctor's opinion, but not to take his medicine.   From the knowledge also that his medicines are given very much at haphazard, the doctor begins to lose faith in his own physic, and is rather pleased than otherwise if the patient neglects to take his prescriptions.   A true faith in medicine is possible only to those who see natural laws of cure. When accurate observation and experience corroborate the exactitude of law, faith in medicine becomes unswerving and perfect.   It is indeed truth that is wanted, and not one-sided advocacy or partial exaggerations.   Not only truth, *but all truth.*

The practical physician who works, often wearily, amongst the sick should rejoice to join hands with the student of nature, who in the same daily experience of disease searches for laws of cure, and watches every opportunity to interrogate nature as to the order of her workings in health and disease.

It is well to know that there is a force in nature often tending towards recovery, well called the " vis medicatrix naturæ,"—well to see that there is method in this force. He that learns this method is the one most likely to aid nature's efforts.

> " Let nature be your teacher ;
> Sweet is the lore which nature brings :
> Our meddling intellect
> Misshapes the beauteous form of things.

> " We murder to dissect ;
> Enough of science and of art,
> Close up those barren leaves :
> Come forth, and bring with you a heart
> That watches and receives."— *Wordsworth.*

In the present time it has become the fashion of extra-scientific physicists and physicians, to sneer at the "vis naturæ," forgetting that there is no more absurdity in recognizing an organic force than an inorganic. The "vis naturæ" is distinctive, although dependent upon and using ordinary inorganic forces, yet ruling them.

Logical-minded as such men are, they forget that it is a castle of their own building they are so intent on casting down.

In an age of imperfect knowledge in the eighteenth century, when the chemical school had done its best and failed, its overthrow was consummated for the time by the physicists and mathematicians who referred all the phenomena of life not to chemical action but to mathematical and physical causes. Alas! their fine reasoning was soon cast to the winds, and the school of Haller put the extinguisher on the pure physicists, again revived in the present day.

It may be answered it is just and reasonable to look for reign of law in science founded on inorganic forces, such as astronomy or physical science, whose phenomena are the most general and invariable, or on chemistry, whose order of facts is more complex. Aye, even the science of organization, physiology, depends on laws, and necessitates order; "but we stop short at therapeutics," cry the physicians. "Here we are satisfied to grope in the dark. We do not search for principles in the forces at work in the diseased human organism when working towards recovery. Enough for us to stand by whilst nature cures *somehow*." To observe nature's method in the cure of disease, and to find out her mode of action, is still as much neglected as in the days of Galen. Hence it is that therapeutics is but a storehouse, truly a rich one, of facts, waiting for the master's hand to show the order of those facts.

CHAPTER V.

THERAPEUTICS.

Knowledge is not a shop for the sale of commodities, but a rich storehouse for the glory of the Creator and the good of mankind.—BACON.

Gross ignorance decries no difficulties: imperfect knowledge finds them out, and struggles with them. It must be perfect knowledge that overcomes them.*

ARE there laws of therapeutics? is a question still asked by medical men. Even one so accurately trained as Dr. James Ross asks the question in the *Practitioner* for January, 1878.

A more important question is, Have laws of therapeutics been discovered? Are we shutting our eyes to the truth, and doing our utmost to obscure the foundations of law in therapeutics?

What a smile of pity would a similar question excite amongst chemists in the present day—Are there laws of definite proportion?—when such laws had already been discovered by Dalton. What a reflection upon the science of therapeutics it is to see Niemeyer, a mind full of practical sagacity, kicking against and refusing to recognize the reign of law in therapeutics; suppos-

---

* Bentham's Principles of Morals and Legislation, vol. ii, chap. xvi, p. 57; quoted in Grote's Plato, vol. i, p. x.

ing himself to be expounding empirical science or the
medicine of experience, yet, unknown to himself, obey-
ing law and showing forth in detail its unchanging
principles!

"In the early stage, he gave a few doses of laudanum, but if the amendment was not rapidly perceptible, he abandoned the opium and had recourse to calomel (a grain every half hour) and *cold* wet packing.
The cold packing especially relieved the sickness, so
much so that patients cried out for the renewal of the
cold as soon as the bandages became at all warm." *
Thus finding the harmony of the law of similars in
prescribing the medicine calomel for catarrhal flux of
the intestines, which has most power to cause flux of
the same surface, and for the deadly coldness of collapse the ice-cold water applications.

Just as absurd as if Faraday refused to acknowledge
Dalton's law of atomic proportion, yet in his life-
work proving the truth of that law under which every
truth of chemistry groups itself. In words refusing to
acknowledge or own all the bounteous store that law
conferred on himself, yet in his life proving that he
was daily a debtor to that law.

Law reigns in nature without governing; obedience
brings abundant fruit. Productiveness becomes the
result of submission; as obedient children, not fashion-
ing ourselves, becomes the highest meed of praise to
the disciple of truth who willingly gives an unsparing

* Niemeyer on the "Symptomatic Treatment of Cholera,"
Practitioner, July 12th, pp. 40, 41.

acknowledgment of the source from whence he derives
help. Alas, that so instructed a man of science as the
late Dr. Anstic should endeavor to obscure the specific
action of ipecacuanha in curing sickness as a "vaso-
motor stimulant," afraid to concede so much to truth
as to acknowledge that this action of the drug is
according to the natural law of similars!

"Dr. Ringer's late work on therapeutics having
asserted the effect of small doses of ipecacuanha in
checking vomiting, the editor wishes to accumulate
evidence upon this matter. But he calls attention to
the fact that should it be proved, as seems likely, that
small doses of ipecacuanha exert a tonic effect upon
the sympathetic system generally, it will be the most
effective blow yet given to the homœopathic theory of
'similia similibus.'"*

"The greatest gap in the science of medicine is to be
found in its final and supreme stage—the stage of
therapeutics. We want to learn distinctly and clearly
what is the action of drugs and of other influences
upon the bodily organs and functions; for every one
nowadays, I imagine, acknowledges that it is only
by controlling or directing the natural forces of the
body, that we can reasonably hope to govern or guide
its diseased actions. Authentic reports of trials with
medicinal substances upon the healthy human body,
must lead at length, tardily perhaps, but surely, to a
better ascertainment of the rules—peradventure to the

---

* The Editor, The Practitioner, vol. iii, p. 281.

discovery even of the laws—by which our practice should be guided."*

"And as to the uses of medicines, with which it is a student's duty to be acquainted, do you not see that the safest guide to a knowledge of their effects upon a disordered body is the knowledge of their effects upon a healthy body?"†

In ordinary works upon "materia medica" and therapeutics, laws of cure are ignored; principles for the selection of medicines are treated as quite secondary. Medicines are classified according to a vague idea of their chief action. Those that act upon the skin, are called diaphoretic; on the kidneys, diuretic; on the bowels, purgatives; those that lessen the heart's action, are called sedative; those which ease pain, anodyne; others are called stimulants, depressants, stomachics, tonics, antiperiodics, etc. This artificial classification effectually destroys the individuality of each medicine.

The chief or predominant action is described as the characteristic of all. This gives a vague uncertainty and hides the special effect. Each medicine has, in fact, a special characteristic or selective action, peculiar to itself, as well as sharing generally in certain properties common to many.

To the student of medicine or to the practitioner, this vagueness of arrangement (it does not deserve the

---

* Sir Thomas Watson, British Medical Journal, January, 1868.

† Dr. King Chambers.

name of classification) is utterly useless and barren. It begets skepticism and haphazard practice. To give medicine to act on the skin or bowels, may be as injurious in one case as beneficial to another. The real question at issue is: What is the principle to guide in the selection of medicinal agents, in the treatment of disease, in what direction does cure lie ; how can I aid the curative process, and how avoid doing mischief? If the Providence of God works by definite curative laws, how can I discover and use *this* knowledge? "Our chief difficulty in comprehending nature is her simplicity—the multitude and boundless variety of results which she educes from one law."*

Each medicine has its own special or individual physiological action on some organ or function of the human body in health. This physiological action is the reflex of the condition of the organ affected.

The physiological action of medicinal agents stands in some positive relationship to its curative action *in disease*. In most cases that relationship is either of similarity or of contrariety. Some few instances seem to stand out, as of no apparent relationship, but they are few, and deeper investigation brings them in amenable to one or the other. Each law has its own way or behavior, so to speak.

Looking to the observation of facts, apart from the theoretic speculations, two primary laws of therapeutics unfold themselves. As Galvani and Faraday have afforded names for Galvanism and Faradism, those two

---

* G. H. Lewis, in Cornhill Magazine, October, 1860, p. 431.

laws of therapeutics may well be called Galen's law, or the antipathic, founded upon the rule of "contraria contrariis," and Hahnemann's, or the homœopathic law, founded upon the relationship of similars.

When the relationship of the medicinal action is contrary to the signs and symptoms of disease, it is necessary to give doses large enough to produce the full physiological or primary action. Such doses must also be frequently repeated, and for a long time, so that by a succession of repressing actions, the disease may be kept suspended or beaten down, as directly the drug action is suspended the diseased activity reappears. Thus the action of bromide of potassium is exactly the opposite to epilepsy. It produces "sleepiness in the daytime, a decided lack of will and of mental activity, dulness of the senses, drooping of the head, considerable weakness of body, and a somnolent tottering gait. Hence it is that the dose must be large enough to produce an evident, though not complete, anæsthesia of the fauces and upper part of the pharynx and larynx." "Small doses are useless: we ought, therefore, particularly in epilepsy, in tetanus, in neuralgia, in reflex paralysis, in angina pectoris, in whooping-cough, to give as large doses as can safely be borne. In affections like tetanus, in which there is an antagonism between the complaint and the remedy, at the same time that we must be giving every hour or every half-hour a fresh dose of the remedy, we must be carefully watching for the disappearance of the symptoms of the nervous affection and their replacement by the symptoms of poisoning by the remedy. In a case of which I know the details, Dr. F. G. succeeded in obtaining the cessation of tetanic symptoms; but, unfortunately, new doses of opium were given after that cessation, and the patient died of poisoning by opium."*

In the treatment of epilepsy by the bromides, to use the words of Brown-Séquard, "The quantity of these medicines to be taken each day must be large enough to produce an evident, though not complete, anæsthesia of the fauces and upper part of the pharynx and larynx, also an acne-like eruption on the face, neck, shoulders, etc."

"It is never safe for a patient to be even only one day without his medicine, so long as he has not been at least fifteen or sixteen months quite free from attacks. Indeed, it is very frequently the case that patients neglecting this rule are seized again with fits after an immunity of several or of many months, one, two, or only a few more days after the interruption of the treatment—in several cases, after an apparent cure of ten, eleven, or twelve months, and in one instance of thirteen months and a few days."

Most of the therapeutic uses of the bromides have a distinct relationship to the physiological action of "contraria contrariis," necessitating the use of large doses frequently repeated; yet in a few cases the relationship is that of "similars," and the small dose is sufficient.

"Such symptoms as sudden numbness, coldness, deadness, or pricking in one or more limbs; sudden distressing, but indefinable feelings in the epigastrium,

---

* Dr. Brown-Séquard, Lancet, March 10, 1866.

abdomen, or hypogastrium, anxiety or fluttering of the heart."

" In such cases the symptoms are due to a derangement of the local circulation, in consequence of a morbid state of the vaso-motor system of nerves. They may be diminished and entirely removed by the use of bromide of potassium in such *moderate* doses as ten or five grains twice or three times daily."*

In a very large experience Dr. McGregor has never been able to cure a single case of epilepsy by bromide of potassium, though he has found it a most valuable agent in the mitigation of the disease.†

Physostigma.—The opposite of strychnia, directly and powerfully diminishes the reflex activity of the spinal cord. As a remedy for tetanus the dose must therefore be continued in increasing quantities until this physiological action is produced, or until the sedative action of the drug is carried to a dangerous extent, or until constant nausea and vomiting compels us to desist.‡

A case of traumatic tetanus is related by Dr. Eben Watson in which physostigma was used. It requires two grains of the alcoholic extract repeated every quarter-hour for three or four doses to produce any good effect. The disease lasted 46 days. For 43 days the physostigma was used, 1026 grains of the alcoholic extract were given, equal to 34 ounces of the powder of the bean.§

---

* Dr. Russell Reynolds, The Practitioner, vol. i, p. 15.
† Edinburgh Medical Review, October, 1869.
‡ Dr. Frazer, The Practitioner. vol. i, p. 86.
§ The Practitioner, vol. iv, p. 210.

CHAPTER VI.

HAHNEMANN'S LAW OF SIMILARS.

THE organ or function upon which a medicine in full doses acts in health is influenced by it when diseased for good or evil, for a longer or shorter time. When the relationship is in the direction of similarity, the diseased organ or function is influenced to expel the disease, as nature does not allow two similar* diseases to exist at the same time in the economy; the action of the medicine, on account of its similarity, searches out the exact seat of disease, and, like a touch of the whip on a sensitive part, it rouses and energizes the organic force, which reacts to expel the diseased action. The medicine whose relationship is similar goes direct to the diseased organ, and expends most of its force on that organ, whereas the action which is dissimilar or antagonistic to the disease expends itself on the entire economy as well as on the diseased portion.

The disease most akin to small-pox is vaccinia, the natural production of which on the people engaged in milking the cows in Gloucestershire was found to render them proof, or nearly so, against the contagion of

---

* " Two fevers cannot exist in the human body at the same time, the stronger arrests or displaces the weaker."—John Hunter.

small-pox. Observing this result, Jenner proposed to use the mild disease, vaccine, as a preventive of the severe disease, small-pox. How simple, but what a precious boon to humanity!*

In this prevention of disease by similarity, Nature may yet show herself more bountiful than man thinks; not a step-mother, as Dr. Haughton calls her.

In 1850 a gentleman from Chelmsford consulted me for his child, aged four years, suffering from eczema. The disease had existed for three years and a half, since the child had been vaccinated, at the age of three months. Soon afterwards a vesicular eruption came out all over the body. This caused the most distressing irritation and suffering to the poor child, especially at night—so much so that the sheets were generally discolored with blood, from the effects of scratching. For the first year she was treated, unsuccessfully, by the family doctor; afterwards, for a time, by a well-known London skin doctor, but without relief. After eighteen months of suffering under ordinary treatment, she was brought to London, and put under the care of a very clever homœopath, who treated her *medicinally* and *dietetically* for nine months, without any relief. The parents then took her to a hydropathic establishment for three months, and subsequently continued the hydropathic treatment at home for four months longer, making free use of the pack, but also without benefit. Then, in despair, they gave up all treatment for a time. Still the poor child got no better, suffering sadly every

* Dr. Anstie, Practitioner.

night from irritation and sleeplessness. The parents then brought her to consult me. After a careful examination into the history of the case and of the treatment, I said to the parents, much to their surprise, that the only mode of cure which seemed to me likely to succeed was homœopathic, but not medicinal ; viz., to *revaccinate the child*—the principle of "similia similibus" suggesting the remedy. I watched for some weeks, in order to find a perfectly healthy infant from whom to procure good vaccine ; then sent for the child, and revaccinated her. On the eighth day after vaccination slight fever came on ; *hundreds of vaccine vesicles* appeared all over the back, shoulders, arms, and chest. Five or six days afterwards they gradually dried up like ordinary vaccine vesicles, and gradually the eczema lessened ; and in the course of three or four weeks, the disease, which had existed for upwards of three and a half years, entirely disappeared, and the child permanently recovered health and strength. The perfect and speedy cure of the child's disease induced the parents at once to have two younger children vaccinated, which up to this they would not allow.*

The action of diuretics is very closely allied to the process at work in certain diseases of the skin. The benefit to be derived from such is well illustrated by Dr. Tilbury Fox.

Mr. George Critchett, in his address at the London Hospital in 1859, said : "The present plan in the treatment of pannus, or vascular opacity of the cornea, the

---

* Lancet, December 18th, 1868.

result of purulent or Egyptian ophthalmia, and the cause of blindness to so many of our soldiers in the East, is to inoculate the eye with purulent matter, and the result in my own practice, as much as in that of others, has been in several instances the recovery of useful sight."*

M., æt. 52, suffered many years from irritating pustules on the face. After revaccination, to my surprise the vaccine pustules on the arm secreted matter freely for three months. The chronic eruption on the face altogether ceased, and did not return, even after the vaccine pustules ceased to discharge.

A lady, aged thirty-two, had suffered for six years from frequently-recurring attacks of painful spasms of the gall-ducts, caused by the passing of inspissated bile and of gall-stones. Many of the attacks ended in temporary jaundice. Year after year she went the round of most of the London physicians distinguished in diseases of the liver, including Dr. Marshall Hall, Dr. Budd, Dr. Burrowes, and many others. Notwithstanding every care in diet, and in the use of various medicines for many years, she continued subject to those frequently-recurring attacks, the cause of which neither medicine, diet, baths, nor exercise seemed able to cure, and nothing to relieve except emetics of ipecacuanha. She consulted me in 1854, and I prescribed various medicines for many months, without benefit. Reflecting on the peculiar condition of the bile and of the gall-ducts, I laid aside all ordinary medicines for a natural

---

* Dr. McCall Anderson, Lancet, November 20th, 1869.

one, and prescribed ten grains of inspissated ox-gall three times a day, three hours after meals. The effect of this was magical : the attacks lessened in frequency, and after a few weeks ceased altogether. For many years she remained perfectly cured.

The simplicity of the means of cure in this case stands out in a most singular relationship to the complexity and variety of medicines which she had used for six years without any relief. Out of a hundred keys there may be one only that will open the lock. In the human frame it is an untold blessing to be enabled promptly to fix upon that one key without trying the ninety and nine—every useless trial more or less injuring the delicate mechanism of the the lock—the fragile human body.

As another illustration. A middle-aged woman had been suffering for many years from the most agonizing attacks of spasms, with vomiting of sour fluid. She had been treated by several doctors with only palliative relief, chiefly by large doses of alkalies, which, however, had no effect on the cure of the cause—the acidity. This returned as badly as ever directly the use of the soda was discontinued. For three years she had also tried ordinary homœopathic medicines, in tincture and globules, without benefit. I prescribed the juice of a lemon in a little water twice a day, about two hours after meals. A three weeks' course of this permanently cured the cause and the result, viz., the acidity and the spasms.

It was the knowledge of the true law of cure which indicated the selection of the remedy.

" Of the actual remedies used for the checking of
the further escape of blood, one of the most important is venesection."   " Herein we are guilty of homœopathy : to prevent bleeding, we draw blood."*

The application of leeches often exerts a specific or
directly curative action in local vascular congestion.

Mrs. ——, aged twenty-six, for five or six years had
frequent miscarriages but no living child.   In 1869 she
suffered much during the course of early pregnancy
from pain over the iliac region and along the course
of the femoral vein, with frequent gushes of blood and
threatenings of miscarriage.   After the application of
four leeches over the right ovarian region the bleeding
ceased, and she went to her full time without a bad
symptom.   To hit upon the exact place to apply leeches
is of great consequence.   If applied to the foot or thigh,
in this case, it would probably have brought on miscarriage—exactly opposite to their effect over the ovarian region.

" *Strychnia in Tetanus.*—We know that strychnia
acts upon the spinal cord, affecting, apparently, those
parts and those functions of the cord which are affected
in tetanus; and in so fatal a malady it would be jus-
tifiable, I conceive, to give the strychnia in the hope
that it might occasion a morbid action which would
supersede the morbid action of the disease, and yet be
less perilous and more manageable than it.   This,
were it successful, would be a cure according to the

---

* Sir Thomas Watson, vol. i, p. 265.

Hahnemannic doctrine—'similia similibus curantur;' a doctrine much older, however, than Hahnemann."*

Dr. Owen Rees, in the *Guy's Hospital Report* for 1855, says that in many cases of alkaline urine with phosphates, he has found an alkaline treatment cure, after the unavailing exhibition of mineral acids.

Dr. King Chambers, in his *Digestion and its Derangements* (p. 173), advises the use of alkalies in cases of acidity, but he says that "if taken before a meal they seem to augment the excess of acid." "In that case," he says, "an exactly opposite course of treatment seems indicated," which he found successful, giving dilute acids to cure the acidity.

Dr. George Johnson's suggestion of the administration of castor oil in cholera, failed because the dose prescribed was too large, and too frequently repeated; a teaspoonful of castor oil every hour was too much even for cholera. The dose, untrue to the laws of similars, from which it was derived, caused the practice to fall into disrepute. The action of castor oil is roughly analogous to the profuse purging of cholera; the frequently repeated large dose left no time for reaction, *i. e.*, cessation of the disease.

Mr. McNamara, who was pupil and house physician under Dr. George Johnson, at King's College Hospital, during the cholera epidemic of 1854, and subsequently had a vast experience of cholera in Calcutta, was predisposed to think well of the eliminative treatment of cholera, and applied it on a large scale

---

* **Sir Thomas Watson.**

with enthusiasm, and on the full understanding of Dr. Johnson's views. He declares that the mortality was frightful, and that he had completely abandoned the method.

Dr. Young, of Florence, is much wiser than Dr. G. Johnson, for he administers castor oil in diarrhœa, in doses of four to six drops.*

From the absence of recognized laws of cure, many most valuable remedies have gone out of use, becoming displaced by new remedies, and finally lost sight of; whereas, if brought into relation with a definite law, the remedy would never have been thus lost sight of. Hydrocyanic acid vapor is a most valuable agent in the treatment of chronic ophthalmia. It sets up a fresh inflammatory action which displaces the old one.

Dr. Turnbull, in his book on *The Use of the Vapor of Hydrocyanic Acid in Diseases of the Eye*, in describing the effect of the vapor in cases of chronic inflammation of the eye, relates that in most cases the

---

* "In Italy acute diarrhœa is one of the commonest affections the physician has to treat. During three years I have made note of upwards of a hundred cases, in patients ranging from three months to seventy years of age, and in more than nine-tenths of the whole, no medicine was used but the (castor oil) emulsion.

"In five typical cases relief was afforded by this oil in periods varying from one to five days.

"I have given it in every form of diarrhœa. When the diarrhœa is chronic, and the stools contain mucus, I usually increase the dose to from four to six drops."—"On the Use of Castor Oil in Diarrhœa," by Dr. Young, of Florence. Practitioner, March, 1875.

vapor excited vascular congestion, increased inflammation of the eye, which lasted for several hours after
each application ; here, in fact, the fresh inflammation
curing the chronic.   A patient of mine (Mr. C——)
suffered for six weeks from a severe attack of iritis, for
which he had been treated by the most powerful applications and medicines without relief.   After a few
applications of the hydrocyanic acid vapor, the affected
eye was perfectly cured.   Delighted with the rapid
cure, he thought that he would improve the vision of
the sound eye by an application of the hydrocyanic
acid vapor.   This brought on a most violent attack of
iritis in the sound eye.

Exophthalmic Goitre.—A young lady (Miss E——),
aged twenty-four, was brought to me in 1850, suffering
from enlargement of the neck, throbbing and distension
of the eyes, which looked as if protruding from their
sockets ; she also complained of distressing headache.
For some months she had been under the care of the
family attendant at Canonbury, who administered
small doses of iodine.   The patient getting no better,
this gentleman took her to the late Sir B. Brodie, who
prescribed large doses of iodide without any relief.
She then consulted Dr. C. J. B. Williams, who prescribed iodide of iron ; this aggravated the headache,
and did not relieve the enlargement of the neck, nor
the distended eyeballs.   She then consulted me ; I
recognized the disease as exophthalmic goitre, from Dr.
Graves's admirable description, although up to that
time I had never treated a case of it.   I knew that
belladonna caused in the healthy human subject, head-

ache, with throbbing in the head and eyes, with vascular excitement. Of this I prescribed four drops of the tincture three times a day. It afforded immediate relief to the headache, gradually lessened the swelling of the neck and the protrusion of the eyes. It was taken regularly for about six weeks, and the cure proved permanent, one of the most satisfactory I ever witnessed. In the treatment of exophthalmic goitre, this case is, I believe, the first case of the successful use of belladonna in that disease. I published this case in the *British Journal of Homœopathy*, vol. xxv, in 1867.

Miss ——, æt. nineteen, suffered for three years, all through the summer, from the worst form of hay asthma, producing sneezing, coryza, redness of the eyes, dyspnœa, with dry wheezing and cough. In the beginning of the summer of 1868 she consulted me. I prescribed arsenic (Fowler's solution), four drops three times a day, with immediate benefit; so much so that she was enabled to live in London (Euston Square) all the summer. The occasional use for three or four days of the arsenic kept her in perfect comfort, although the previous three years she found no relief till she went to the seaside.

Dr. Copland, in his *Dictionary of Practical Medicine*, narrates a most instructive case. Being summoned to a young lady who had suffered for twenty-four hours from violent palpitation of heart, to the surprise of the parents he prescribed a cup of the strongest green tea, which, in a person in health, easily excites palpitation. It speedily relieved her.

December, 1861.—A gentleman called on me, having suffered for a fortnight with most distressing irritation of the neck of the bladder, night and day, causing constantly recurring painful micturition. For a fortnight he had been taking full doses of bicarbonate of potash with tincture of henbane, without relief. I prescribed ten drops of pure tincture of cantharides in six ounces of water, one-sixth part every four hours. The first dose relieved, and two days' use of it perfectly cured him.

Another case illustrates the specific action of cantharis. A gentleman, aged forty-four, living near Liverpool, had suffered for four days from total suppression of urine, notwithstanding the use of hot baths, hot fomentations, and various medicines prescribed by two local doctors. Not a drop of urine was secreted till five drops of strong tincture of cantharides was administered on the fourth day by his young brother, my assistant. Within half an hour, urine began to flow, and after a second dose of the same, the secretion was gradually restored. The knowledge of direct therapeutical laws placed the youth in a position, as far as the patient's welfare was concerned, far ahead of those two "experienced" medical men. What a boon to humanity thus to be saved from losing time in trying indirect means! It brings remedies into the condition of positive agents, to search out the diseased organ, and to rouse the suspended or vitiated functions.

" While the discharge of gleet is whitish or opaque, two or three drops of copaiba in frequent doses is often useful; and when the prostate has lost its tenderness if pressed by the finger, one or two drops of tincture of cantharides, in plain water, four times in twenty-four hours, is also sometimes magical in its effect."*

A lady suffered from total obstruction of the bowels for upwards of a month. After the unavailing use of injections and of purgatives, including croton oil, the obstruction yielded to a large dose—three grains of acetate of lead with as much calomel, and one grain of opium, prescribed by an old country doctor. In a case of obstruction of the bowels of fifteen days' duration, I prescribed one grain of acetate of lead in a tablespoonful of distilled water. Within eight hours free evacuation of the lower bowel followed, although injections, strong purgatives, and galvanism had failed to relieve. The cause of the obstruction being a scirrhous tumor, the relief was but temporary.

In mental diseases the knowledge of "similia similibus" is of signal use. For vicious habits or destructiveness do not substitute a killing torpor, rather fresh activity and healthy pursuits. Goethe, in *Wilhelm Meister*, describes an old physician highly successful in the cure of mental diseases, whose principle it was to fix upon the morbidly active tendency of each patient, and give that tendency incessant occupation, so as to use up the nerve-force, that, allowed to accumulate, only irritated mind and body.

A singular case was related some years ago in one of the journals, by the physician of a lunatic asylum. One patient, most dangerously violent, destroyed every

---

* Lancet, February 12th, 1875.

particle of grass in the garden, eating it all! Taking
the hint from this, the doctor supplied the patient with
an unlimited quantity of green vegetables. This proved
the main agent in his cure. This case is a beautiful
illustration of what a marvellous power the laws of
cure become to the true physician, alive to every possible application of the laws, suggesting many things—
baths, external applications, diet, exercise, moral management—which might not enter the mind without the
prompting of law. Then, indeed, the physician finds
that the truest direction of cure is to get out of the attitude of antagonism to nature.

Brain-force becomes morbid through idleness, often
" vents itself" on the mucous membrane of the stomach and bowels—simulating diarrhœa or dysentery.
A youth, about eleven, was brought to me, having
suffered from chronic dysentery for a year. Looking
at the large head, active temperament, and irritable,
restless manner of the boy, I asked the father if the
boy went to school? " Oh, no!" said the father, "all
the lessons are laid aside, and he has had every opportunity of careful treatment, yet he gets no better." To
which I answered, " It is hard work and occupation
the boy wants, and not rest and coddling." A few
weeks' daily use of gymnastics perfectly cured what a
year's medication failed to do.

Mr. George Combe, in his work on *America* narrates his visiting a physician, who lamented to him
most piteously the sad conduct of his apprentice, who
had broken almost every window and door in the house,
from morning to night destroying something, hinges

or locks, doors or windows; that he tried every means of correction, flogging and starving, but all in vain. Looking at the large active brain of the boy, a happy thought suggested itself,—to use strong exercise to cure the boy's destructiveness. Accordingly, the next morning, the doctor got up at six o'clock, took the boy to the wood-house, and gave him all the wood for the day's use to cut up. At this he worked most cheerfully. For the first day during his apprenticeship there was no mischief done. The brisk exercise made him so happy that he no longer needed the doctor to call him, but regularly every morning cut up enough wood for the day's consumption, and never again gave his master any trouble.

Dr. George Johnson, in one of his lectures upon overwork of the mind, from distress and anxiety, says: "It is not without interest to remark that in many cases we can cure those patients of their bad dreams, and of their drowsiness, by giving an opiate at bedtime for a few nights in succession."

The Influence of a Suit of Clothes.—A refractory patient at Colney Hatch was in the habit of tearing his clothes into shreds. Mr. Tyerman, one of the medical officers, ordered him to be dressed in a bran new suit. The poor man, a tailor by trade, either from a professional appreciation of the value of his new habiliments, or from being touched by this mark of attention, respected their integrity, and from that moment rapidly recovered. Before leaving the asylum, he stated that he owed his cure to the good effect produced upon his mind by being intrusted with this new suit of clothes.

In the *Times* newspaper of June 17th, 1856, a painful case is related. An old pauper lunatic became quarrelsome, and struck the doctor of the asylum. For this the unfortunate man was punished by a cold shower-bath for half an hour, and a powerful dose of tartar emetic, a few minutes after which he died. When the surgeon and three or four attendants were forcing the poor unhappy creature into the dreaded cold shower-bath, he begged piteously to be "sent to work on the farm" in place of the cold shower-bath.

How natural it would have been to cure the old man's violence by hard work rather than cause his death by 600 gallons of cold water showered down upon his head in twenty-eight minutes.

"Give the patient a draught made from the root of mandrake in a smaller dose than will induce mania." This in order to cure mania.*

Let us not forget that our success depends very much on going with, and not thwarting or destroying, the "vis medicatrix naturæ;" the true physician is ready to ascribe a due credit to nature as well as to art, the handmaiden of nature. In the end all exaggeration defeats itself. It is absurd to ascribe all our success to our treatment, or to ignore the natural force in the organism which struggles to right itself. The truest confidence comes from an open, honest study of what nature can do, and of what she cannot do.

Laws of therapeutics keep before the doctor's mind all true curative actions, tell when it is safe abruptly to arrest disease, and at times they indicate that to cure

---

* Hippocrates.

quickly may set up a far greater evil than the original disease. A gentleman living at Saffron Waldon had been for years subject to humid asthma, aggravated by a soft polypus in the nose. This for several years secreted such an amount of mucus that he was accustomed to use five or six pocket-handkerchiefs a day. Two celebrated London surgeons at different times tried to extract the polypus, but, fortunately for the patient, only succeeded in tearing away a part. The polypus continued to secrete freely; as long as it did so his general health continued good. Some time afterwards the polypus grew backwards, pressing upon the soft palate, and produced discomfort in swallowing. Much annoyed with this, on a visit to a friend at Manchester, he called on a well-known surgeon there. This gentleman, in his consulting-room, without any preparation whatever, passed a ligature round the polypus, and removed the entire mass. The profuse discharge from the nose that had existed for years disappeared at once. Slight congestion of the brain came on a few days afterwards. This gradually increased for a week or ten days, and resulted in paralysis (hemiplegia of the right side). A few weeks after the operation he returned from Manchester, and consulted me for the paralysis. The nose was still perfectly dry. I tried to set up a fresh discharge by the use of iodide of potassium, of snuff, and hot-water fomentations, etc. ; all, however, to no purpose, as the paralysis slowly increased, and ended in death two years after the total arrest of the copious secretion from the nose.

What a boon if the surgeon had recognized the necessity, after suddenly putting an end to such a profuse
secretion, to set up another discharge for a time.   If
he had suggested the use of ordinary snuff or of a
seidlitz powder every morning for a few weeks after
the removal of the polypus, the operation might have
proved a blessing to the poor man, whereas it embit-
tered the remaining years of his life.

CHAPTER VII.

GALEN'S LAW—THE ANTIPATHIC.

REJOICING to enlarge the boundaries of knowledge, true science cannot ignore any law, though its sphere of action be limited and not of universal application. Galen's law of "contraria contrariis" has its place, and a very prominent place, still in the practice of every physician. The therapeutic action of certain medicines seems to lie altogether, or nearly so, in that direction— such as the bromide of potassium in epilepsy, sleep- lessness, with dreaming, nervous excitement, hysteria, spasms. These are symptoms exactly opposite to the drug action, which proves invaluable in such cases, and not to be despised, although it is but a temporary action requiring frequent repetition and long con- tinuance.

Nothing can be more unsatisfactory than the disap- pointment felt by doctors and patients in the application of chemical remedies according to Galen's law of "contraria contrariis." Undoubtedly the use of alka- lies relieves acidity ; but the relief is, alas, but tempo- rary and evanescent. It is the illustration of a true palliative, i. e., a medicine of short action, relieving for a little time, and then allowing the old symptoms to re- turn, same or worse than ever. Even after a full course of the natural alkaline water at Vichy, I have known patients lose the gravel during their stay there, which returned as badly as ever a few days after leaving Vichy. The larger the experience the more disappointing in permanent results is the use of alkalies in acidity, whether of stomach, of blood, of perspiration, or of urine. Not to underrate the temporary palliation, for many a case of calculi in the kidney or ureters, the only temporary comfort is to be had from small doses of alkalies in a large quantity of water. When cure is not possible, palliation is to be welcomed, even at the disadvantage of keeping up the use of the remedy for months or years.*

A dissimilar action may suspend a disease for a time, but seldom cures permanently. I observed epilepsy to be arrested in two cases by the occurrence of porrigo. As soon as the latter was cured, the epilepsy returned as badly as ever. If mania occur in a consumptive patient, the lung symptoms are often arrested till the

---

* The phenomena of gout correspond closely to the doctrine of elimination, as from first to last a preservative effort of the economy. Nature is not invariably a " step-mother," as Dr. Haughton rather harshly described her. From anxiety of mind, errors in diet, want of exercise, or from imperfect work of kidneys, as in lead-poisoning or Bright's disease, the food becomes imperfectly assimilated. An excess of uric acid accumulates in the blood, which disturbs and oppresses the various organs of the body. Nature or the organic force reacts to expel this poison, and deposits the uric acid as urate of soda upon the structures of the joints and tendons which have the least complex structure, and whose chemical activity is stronger than the organic.

mania passes off, when they return with increased
force.

Belladonna in Salivation.—A woman, treated by
mercury internally and externally for serious diarrhœa,
was affected with profuse salivation. Dr. Erpenbeck
treated this latter complaint with belladonna in divided
doses of 2½ grains taken in emulsion every twenty-four
hours. Next day the salivation had subsided, and the
mouth was dry. On stopping the belladonna the salivation returned, and again ceased when it was resumed.*

The action of purgatives is dissimilar to disease of
the skin, hence the unsatisfactory result of such treatment. "For no one who has carefully studied eczema
can have failed to observe the injury which usually
follows upon a long course of purgatives. . . . It is
true that during their use the eruption may improve
or disappear; but whenever they are stopped, it flour-
ishes again as luxuriantly as ever, while the debility is
immeasurably increased."†

In Dr. Copland's *Dictionary of Practical Medicine*,
an instructive case of acute rheumatism is related,
where a full dose of croton oil was administered in the
hope of cutting short the disease. The most violent
purging came on and killed the patient in twenty-four
hours, without any relief whatever to the rheumatic
pains.

Two dissimilar actions frequently coexist, the disease and the medical action contrary to it; hence it is

---

* Hanover Correspondence Blatt.
† Dr. McCall Anderson, p. 66.

10

that cure does not follow, although the disease is held
in check for a short time, springing up with activity
again the instant the action of the medicine is suspended.
A dissimilar disease has the power only to suspend the
other; when the more active runs its course, the other
shows itself. The full physiological action of a drug
(medicine) has the same mode of behavior as disease.
The antipathic action of medicines touches the exact
seat of the disease, or the diseased point in the organism, in a way opposite to the disease, when reaction ensues; it is the same diseased action which recurs.

A case of urticaria complicating small-pox occurred
at the Hôpital Beaujon in Paris in October, 1869, under
the care of M. Gubler. The patient was a non-vacci-
nated female, who, on the third day of a variolous eruption of a severe character, became covered with urticaria, attended by intense pruritus. This lasted three
days, during which the variolous eruption remained
stationary. Variola then resumed its course, and the
patient eventually rallied, notwithstanding such bad
symptoms as epistaxis, etc.

The physiological action of iodide of potassium is
akin to the ulceration of the mucous membrane of the
nose and throat. It is much less analogous to the deepseated tertiary symptoms, such as disease of the liver or
of the coats of bloodvessels. In such, even when
given in large doses, it seldom cures, but gives the
most signal temporary relief; after a time the disease
reappearing, to be again beaten down by the same
medicine. By a succession of palliative actions cure
may result, the disease getting weaker after each

palliation.   Such indirect cure is slower and less effectual than when the direct specific action of medicine is applicable.

A papular eruption suspends a vesicular—but does not cure it—as the vesicular vaccinia does the similar eruption, small-pox.   Two children suffering from eczema, contracted measles—the eczema vanished during the measles, but after the latter had run its course, the eczema—non-analogous disease—returned as bad as ever.*

Measles generally suspends vaccine and small-pox (a dry, papular eruption, dissimilar to the moist eruption).   After the measles passed away, the vaccine resumed its course, and on the seventeenth day looked like what it usually does on the tenth.*

A lady in the last stage of phthisis, with fatty disease of the liver, was suffering from chronic diarrhœa. For this a London physician prescribed decoction of logwood, which quickly stopped the diarrhœa, but caused sickness and the most intolerable distress from offensive, greasy perspirations, making the room smell day and night as a room does just after a candle is blown out. This proved so annoying that she sent for me, wishing to have anything done that would remove the offensive perspirations. I prescribed small doses of mercury, which reproduced the diarrhœa, put an end to the loathsome perspiration, and relieved the sickness.

In acute rheumatism, with effusion into the joints, the action of blisters over or near the seat of disease,

---

* Hahnemann's Organon, p. 137.

as recommended by Dr. H. Davis, is most useful, because the action of the blister is akin to the inflammation of the synovial membrane of the joint when inflammatory action is intense. But in the relationship of contrary, "blisters are not suited to cases of acute rheumatism in which there is not much inflammatory swelling, although the pain and intolerance of movement be very great."

The receptivity to analogous irritation is increased in disease. This is a fact easily proved : a teaspoonful of castor oil will freely purge a patient suffering from diarrhœa ; yet when constipation exists, the same individual will probably require a tablespoonful to produce the purgative action. When the reflex irritability of the spine is increased, as in tetanus, a most minute dose of strychnia, $\frac{1}{200}$th of a grain, will increase that irritability, and bring on muscular jerking, whereas it would require $\frac{1}{20}$th of a grain to bring on jerking in the natural state of spine of the same individual.

Sir Thomas Watson writing of the use of strychnia in tetanus says: "If the dose be too large, a temporary* aggravation of the disease may show itself for a short time."

An adult person in health would require twenty grains of ipecacuanha to cause sickness ; a patient suffering from nausea would require about two grains to bring on vomiting, but half a grain or less would probably cure the nausea altogether—quickly displacing the nausea without causing sickness.

---

* Often a good sign that the medicine has gone straight home to the disease.

A moderate dose, *i.e.*, less than sufficient to produce the full physiological action, suffices by similarity of action to displace and overcome the disease to which it is akin. From such there is a reaction towards health, *i. e.*, contrary to the disease. If the dose is too strong, the reaction may be too violent. If the dose is too small, it is useless.

A gentleman, A. S., suffered for upwards of a year from sciatica; the pain he described, was an aching *numbness* along the course of the sciatic nerve. He had used medicines internally and externally for a year, baths of various sorts, galvanism, without any but temporary relief. I prescribed four drops of tincture of aconite three times a day. After three days there was no appreciable relief, when the dose was increased to six drops, yet without result. Satisfied with the essential relationship of the numbness which aconite always produces to the numbness of his sciatica, I ordered him to increase the dose to seven drops. This quickly and permanently cured this disease of upwards of a year's duration. "About half an hour after I took the seven drops," the patient said, "a peculiar thrill shot into the thigh and leg of that side *increasing the numbness.*" He took two doses more, of seven drops each, and was perfectly cured; thus, although the relationship of the medicine was similar to the disease, the small dose was insufficient to cure.

The dose, in fact, in similarity must be moderate, less than the dose which produces the full physiological effects, still not too small or it may prove useless.*

Medical men find that patients and their friends are singularly acute nowadays.   In the treatment of a case of chorea in private practice, directly the father found out that the prescribed dose of hemlock was as nearly as could be to a poisonous one, he would seek for another physician accustomed to cure chorea without semi-poisonous† doses of strong medicines.   If a powerful medicine is given in large doses, frequently repeated for a long time, there is a decided risk of causing disease of the organ on which it specially acts.   Thus the enormous doses of succus conii might lay the foundation of paralysis of motion ; a little stronger dose might produce death.   I question if Socrates drank as much hemlock juice at the hands of the executioner of justice as the child described by Dr. John Harley.‡

Dr. John Harley on Conium in the Treatment of Chorea.—Jane R., aged 12, a delicate girl.   ℥ij succus conii gradually increased to ℥iii.   It invariably produced giddiness, heaviness, as if from an inclination to

---

* In scores of cases I have found the same, *i. e.*, a disease to be quickly cured by cautiously increasing the dose, but not changing the remedy when well selected.

† Most practitioners will regard the circumstance that the succus conii effects a cure in chorea only after four or five pints of it have been imbibed as rather a cogent reason for eschewing it altogether, or at least for at once casting about for another and a better remedy.—Dr. Berry, Practitioner, vol. iii, p. 283.

‡ The Practitioner, vol. i, p. 141.

sleep, and dulness. She was not, however, allowed to give way to these feelings, but kept in active motion.

A. V. aged 12 years. Succus conii, ʒiv ter diem for seven days; "each dose made him very giddy, and nearly took him off his legs."

"The jailer handed the cup (of hemlock-juice) to Socrates and said, 'You have only to walk about till your legs are heavy, and then to lie down, and the poison will act.' . . . . A while after drinking the poison the man pressed his foot hard, and asked him if he could feel; and he said 'No,' and then his legs, and so upwards, and showed us that he was cold and stiff."*

James R., aged 6 years, a slender boy. For 18 days took ʒiv gs. bis diem succus conii, then for 14 days longer ʒvi thrice a day; each dose produced a decided effect. A quarter of an hour afterwards he was obliged to lie down.

Thus for 90 days the child was kept on the verge of poisoning for the cure of a disease like chorea that one-third of that number of days of gymnastics would have cured.

The gymnastic master at the Paris Hôpital des Enfants cured twenty such cases by open-air gymnastics in a few weeks.

The doctor accustomed to trust much to the anti-pathic action of large doses persevered with for a long time is apt to get discouraged at his want of success in the actual cure of disease. He gets dissatisfied too

---

* Plato's Phaedo, p. 467, Professor Jowett's translation.

with the evil after-effects of medicines antagonistic to the disease. Thus to a patient in phthisis the use of morphia to still the irritating cough, causes depression of spirits, want of appetite, and headache; the most undesirable effects that can be produced.* In such cases I have for twenty years past prescribed, with the most signal relief, the inhalation of five to ten drops of tincture of iodine,† from a jug of boiling water, for five minutes at bedtime. The relief is most effectual, and unattended by the miserable after-effects of the morphia the next day.

In many cases, when a special effect must be produced for a special purpose, the medical man has to produce the full physiological action of a drug directly contrary to the state of the organ or function affected. Atropia to dilate the pupil in iritis, ergot of rye to arrest uterine haemorrhage or expedite delivery, purgatives to overcome obstruction of the bowels, iodide of potassium in tertiary syphilis; thus the amount of dose is subject to accurate demonstration. Setting out from the primary laws of similarity or contrariety, the regulation of the doses of medicine becomes an accurate induction. If the relationship of the medicinal effects be analogous to the symptoms of the disease, the increased sensibility which this law of action begets calls for a moderate dose, i.e., less than the amount required to produce the full physiological effects.

When the relationship is opposite or dissimilar to

---

* The bad action of a drug.—Brown Séquard.

† The primary action of which is to cause irritation of the larynx and bronchial tubes.

the symptoms of the disease, then full (large) doses are required, and more frequent repetition.

The subcutaneous injection of medicines has introduced increased accuracy of the knowledge of physiological action of medicines, and enables us to use a smaller dose than necessary for administration by the mouth. It would seem also to enable us to reach the nervous system much more completely without disturbing the general system to the same degree as if the full dose were administered by the mouth. It has the great disadvantage for a chronic case, that each dose requires a visit.

The cause of disease is often subtle, finely divided, as when a few minutes' exposure to the infection of typhus or scarlatina engenders the disease; or for a long time, as when residence in a malarious district leads to ague. In like manner the continuous action of minute quantities of a highly divided substance, like the vapor of iodine, may cure disease in a most satisfactory way. A lady, aged 40, suffered from induration and enlargement of the liver, which after resisting all medical treatment for some months, was perfectly and permanently cured in a few weeks by the vapor arising from an ounce of pure crude iodine exposed in a dish all night in her bedroom. Every particle of the iodine disappeared in vapor during the month. The induration and enlargement gradually diminished, and her health was permanently restored.

Remedies seem to vary in their adaptability for cure; thus most of the uses of bromide of potassium

are very distinctly in a relationship of "contrary" to
its effects on the healthy human body, whereas all or
most of the uses of arsenic are in the relationship of
"similar."*

---

* See note on p. 93.

CHAPTER VIII.

THE LAW OF SIMILARS ALONGSIDE THE LAW OF CONTRARIES.

THE modern chemical school of physicians have scarcely got a step farther in therapeutic science than their predecessors of the sixteenth century. As yet they have no principle beyond that of Galen's—for acidity give alkalies, for alkalinity give acids. Yet the experience of all medical men shows that such prescribing is but palliative, and seldom if ever curative.*

---

* " First of all, let me speak of the general principles upon which the treatment should be conducted. A very simple rule —indeed, too simple, I think—is often adopted. When the urine has persistently and habitually thrown down acid deposits, the patient has generally been prescribed alkalies; if, on the contrary, he has had alkaline deposits, he has been treated with acids. That simple mode has too often formed the main portion of the treatment. In the former case he has soda or potash largely administered, or he will be told to drink so many glasses of Vichy water, which is mainly a strong solution of carbonate of soda, only a natural instead of an artificial one. Now it is quite true that with alkalies, provided enough be taken, these deposits will disappear ; the uric acid will no longer be deposited ; the urine will become less irritating ; the annoying symptoms will be diminished or got rid of. And of course the patient is very much pleased with this new condition of clear urine and disappearance of all deposit. And you will say, ' What

Nitric Acid in Lithic Acid Gravel.—Lady B., æt. 78, suffered for five months from uric acid gravel, which caused great agony at each act of urination. She was treated by her doctor at Scarborough with large quantities of Vichy water, without benefit. She was then removed to her daughter's house in London, who sent for Dr. Garrod. He prescribed large doses of alkalies, and, to mitigate the great pain, two or three doses of morphia each day. Thus for a week she lived half the day free from pain, and then utterly wretched from the sickness after the morphia, the pain worse than ever till the next dose. Her daughter then sent for me. The old lady was moaning most piteously, sick and unable to touch food after the morphia. The urine was pale, highly acid, contained much uric acid gravel, causing urination with much strangury.

---

more can be desired ?' This : you have merely made his enemy disappear, but he is by no means rid of its presence ; you have not checked the acid formation. The uric acid is there as ever ; but the uric acid and the urates are soluble in alkali, and you have only made them invisible. You really have the same condition as that of the fabled ostrich, which is said to put its head in the bush when pursued by hunters, and, no longer seeing them, believes itself secure. Just such is the security of the patient with uric acid who trusts solely to alkalies or Vichy water. His surplus deposits have become imperceptible to *his* vision ; nothing more. I do not say that the alkalies have been absolutely unserviceable as regarding his constitutional state, but they will not improve it to any great extent ; and when he leaves them off the acid shows itself again."—Clinical Lecture on the Early History of Calculous Disease, and the Treatment best adapted for its Prevention. By Sir Henry Thompson, F.R.C.S., etc. From the Lancet of January 13th, 1872.

I prescribed ten drops of dilute nitric acid in half a tumbler of water four times a day. It afforded immediate and permanent relief. Within twenty-four hours it caused the urine to become dark-colored, with a copious deposit of urate of ammonia. The uric acid disappeared, and the dark, dense, muddy urine, to her surprise, caused no pain. The pale acid urine, full of crystals, having been touched by the magic alchemy of its analogue, was broken up and made innocuous.

The old lady used to smile with intense satisfaction, mixed with a certain suspicion that it was some sort of witchcraft that so soon relieved her of all pain and sickness, restored her appetite, and enabled her to sleep without morphia.

Mr. ——, living in Ryde, consulted me in 1865 for advanced granular degeneration of the kidneys, accompanying chronic gout. The feet were œdematous; he was thin and exhausted, suffering from frequent attacks of gout in the hands and feet.

The urine was abundant, pale; low specific gravity, 1010; contained albumen in moderate quantity; under the microscope it contained numberless crystals of lithic acid and granular casts. The disease had existed for three or four years. I prescribed dilute nitric acid, seven or eight drops in a wineglass of water three or four times a day. It had a most striking effect. The attacks of gout became much less frequent; the urine got darker and of higher specific gravity. All the symptoms of urea-poisoning passed off, and the dropsy. His health became much restored for some years, although eventually the kidney disease progressed towards a fatal termination.

Master B., æt. 4, for upwards of a year suffered from irritation of the bladder with incontinence of urine caused by lithic acid gravel in the urine. I prescribed dilute nitric acid, four drops in a wineglass of water three times a day. In a few weeks the incontinence of urine disappeared as the action of the mineral acid arrested or displaced the formation of the organic (the lithic) acid.

The effect of the nitric acid on the gravel was immediate and most marked, the more so as alkali (the free use of Vals water) had failed to relieve.

The cure was permanent for a year, after that a slight recurrence yielded to a week's use of the same remedy.

Master F., æt. 3, brought to me from Barnet in a low prostrate condition, for many months suffering from pain and difficulty in passing urine, which was scanty, pale, highly acid, with a copious deposit of lithic acid crystals. His appetite was bad, tongue pasty and white. Alkalies in various forms had been tried, including the use of Ems water, Vichy water, Carlsbad water. Their effect was to destroy the little appetite the child had, although not relieving the bladder distress.

I prescribed dilute nitric acid, three drops in half a wineglass of water three times a day half an hour before meals. It immediately restored the appetite, and freshened up the dull, weary-looking child.

After ten days' use of it the urine became darker

colored, the crystals of lithic acid disappeared, and the
child was restored to good health.

A young man, a house-surgeon at Guy's Hospital,
after a long period of incessant study, was seized with
epileptoid convulsions, especially affecting the right
side of the head and face, with stiffness of the neck, of
the lower jaws, and of the tongue. For a day or two
he was treated at the hospital; unrelieved he was removed to his father's house at Muswell Hill, and for
four days most kindly attended by one of the assistant
physicians of the hospital, treated with purgatives,
calomel, cold lotions to the head, and a variety of indirect means, without *any relief to the convulsions*, which
became more and more frequent and severe. On the
fourth day the doctor proposed bleeding, saying he
feared inflammation of the brain. The father of the
young man refused to permit this, asked the doctor
from the hospital to retire, and sent for me. I found
the patient in a state of distressing excitement, with
heavy oppressive headache, stiffness of the neck, of the
lower jaw, and of the tongue, and soft but frequent
pulse. For four nights he had been sleepless from the
frequently recurring spasms. I prescribed five drops
every two hours of tincture of ignatia, which in full
doses in the healthy human body produces "headache,
with heaviness of the forehead; sleeplessness, with
sudden startings which prevent sleep; convulsive muscular spasms with stiffness."*

After three doses the convulsive tendency was ar-

* Hahnemann's Materia Medica Pura, vol. ii, p. 167.

rested, and the young man felt complete relief from the distressing headache and stiffness of the neck. Natural sleep followed, and in a few days he was up and out. To find the specific (ignatia) was to find the only key that fitted and could unlock the jewel-case, whilst the indirect means, the purgatives, cold lotions, etc., were like the chisel and the hammer, which could hack and hew the jewel-case but not open the lock.

Acute Nephritis of four months' duration, with Albuminuria and Hæmaturia, cured by small doses of Turpentine and the use of Hot-air Baths.—Master S., æt. 14, was at school in November, 1866, when scarlatina broke out. He had all the symptoms of scarlatina, but no eruption. He was soon afterwards sent home to his father's house in Devonport, and for ten days seemed languid and feverish, with all the symptoms of scarlatina but no eruption. He remained for some weeks under the care of the family doctor, but recovered so far as to be able to go to the same school, January 30th, 1867. Some weeks after that date he was again complaining of loss of appetite, great depression, and swelling of the eyelids. He continued ill till he was sent home again, April 18th. Pains in the limbs and back came on, with great prostration, sickness, swelling of the legs and feet. He continued in this state, attended by the family doctor, for five weeks. The latter urged him to be taken to London and placed under the care of Dr. George Johnson. He attended him closely for ten days, prescribed large doses of citrate of magnesia and broom tea; subsequently perchloride of iron, occasionally a warm-water bath. Every day he got worse. Each dose of the medicines caused vomiting, so that he lay in a state of torpor, unable to take food, the appetite quite gone. The doctor looked gloomy, and gave no hopes of recovery, as he saw the patient sinking deeper and deeper into a heavy state of comatose stupor.

In an agony of distress, the mother asked Dr. G. Johnson to retire from the case, and sent for me. I found the patient propped up in bed with a number of pillows, nearly suffocating with œdema of the lungs, the eyelids closed by œdema, which extended from the forehead to the feet. He slept day and night in a low stupor; with difficulty could he answer a question, utterly refusing food. The urine was abundant, absolutely thick with blood. It contained so much albumen that on boiling it became quite solid in the test-tube.

The diseased condition seemed to me exactly the analogue of the physiological action of turpentine.*

It was given in the dose of four drops every two hours in a teaspoonful of water. At once, also, I administered a hot-air bath in the bed, by means of a large spirit-lamp under the bed-clothes, held up by hoops in the shape of a tent over his body. After half an hour of the spirit-lamp, the blankets becoming very hot were closely packed round his body. Profuse

---

* "Two persons who had used turpentine improperly for several days (one for gravel, the other for tapeworm) were affected for upwards of a fortnight with albuminuria, blood having been freely passed, and some fibrinous blood-casts; and the irritation of the kidney was intense."—Dr. Heywood Thompson, Lancet, July 4th, 1857.

perspiration followed, which continued day and night for forty-eight hours. In twenty-four hours the unconsciousness passed away. The sickness ceased on the third day of treatment, and the appetite gradually returned. The turpentine was given at less frequent intervals for a month. The quantity of blood gradually lessened, and the dropsy was carried off. The patient rapidly recovered health and strength. The albumen perfectly disappeared in six weeks, and the kidneys have continued ever since perfectly sound, although the disease had existed for four to five months.

The direct or specific action of the turpentine touched curatively the diseased structure of the kidneys. It set up a new action similar to the diseased action. As a result the economy received a curative impulse that showed itself so clearly as to enable us to speak with confidence of perfect restoration at the time when the orthodox doctor could see nothing but death in the case. His indirect treatment, the magnesia, broom tea, and iron, had no "good action," in the graphic words of Brown-Séquard. It had a most palpable bad action, utterly disgusting the stomach with food, and allowing the dropsy to invade the lungs. The warm-water bath prostrated the patient without inducing perspiration. The spirit-lamp bath, *used in bed*, caused no exertion to the patient, and set up the most profuse perspiration. In a case of actual life and death such as this, the indirect action of the bath should be prompt and decided, or else not used at all.

General Dropsy, dependent on Degeneration (probably granular) of the Kidney, cured by small doses of

Turpentine.—Captain S., æt. 59. Bilious temperament, deep sallow complexion, and of a family in which kidney disease carried off several members at his age. Given up as hopeless by the ordinary physicians in the country, he was with difficulty moved to his mother-in-law's house at Croom's Hill, Greenwich, and placed under my care. The morning after his arrival I found him after a night of much suffering, propped up in bed, scarcely able to breathe, with his legs and body œdematous, the entire posterior inferior region of the right side of chest perfectly dull on percussion, and in the upper and middle parts moist crepitating râles; the same on the left side, but to a slighter extent; the heart's action muffled and indistinct. On the least exertion, even in bed, sudden faintness or oppression of breathing came on. His tongue was dry and red, and the bowels constipated; no appetite; extreme prostration of strength, and lassitude. The urine was abundant (three to four pints in the twenty-four hours), of a pale color, specific gravity 1010, reaction neutral, freely coagulated by boiling; under the microscope, broken-down blood-disks were seen entangled in casts of the tubuli uriniferi and epithelial scales. The history given me was that his constitution had been severely tried in India and at home by enormous quantities of calomel and by various accidental falls; that for years past he was accustomed to pass bloody urine. In January, after a severe kick on the loins from his horse, bloody urine was passed, with severe aching pain across the loins. He was confined to his house, under the care of two local practitioners, for four months, during which dropsy gradually came on and steadily increased, notwithstanding the most vigorous treatment, including the free use of calomel and of warm baths.

I prescribed turpentine in five-drop doses every three hours. This dose causing bilious diarrhœa, it was lessened to two drops, and continued for three months with the most rapid improvement. The dropsy was gradually removed; the breathing was relieved, appetite and strength increased, bowels acted regularly once a day; and about the 28th of June he returned home, to the astonishment of his former medical attendants and friends, as well able to walk as ever, and in perfect health. In May, 1855, he called on me in London, and reported "that he had continued in perfect health, able to hunt and to go about in the coldest weather, till about a fortnight ago, when, the stomach getting deranged, he had foolishly allowed his old surgeon to give him smart doses of calomel for a few days, which upset his general health, and his limbs became a little swollen again." Under the terebinthina, two drops night and morning for ten days, he became again quite restored to his usual activity and strength.

The cure in this case was not permanent. Upon careful examination a year afterwards, I found the urine to contain a little albumen, the specific gravity 1012. Some months afterwards he took cold, with symptoms of pleurisy. The country doctor bled him, and in a few days he died.

Acute Nephritis with Albuminuria, General Dropsy of eight months' duration, cured by large doses of Turpentine when small doses failed.—Miss ——, æt. 26, of a feeble constitution, lymphatic temperament, in March, during the prevalence of cold east winds, was attacked by severe pain across the lumbar region, accompanied with the secretion of thick white urine. Anasarca came on in June, with great prostration of strength. Under ordinary (allopathic) treatment she became gradually worse till the following November, when she was placed under my care. Her limbs were then enormously swollen, deeply pitting on pressure; the integument of the body and chest also universally anasarcous. She complained of much muscular weakness, but her appetite was good. Bowels regular; catamenia absent four months. The urine—32 oz. in the twenty-four hours—of a smoky, opalescent color; specific gravity 1018. On boiling, it became a nearly solid mass of albumen. Under the microscope numerous blood-globules were visible. I prescribed five drops of turpentine four times a day. After a week's use of this, finding she was no better, I increased the dose to ten drops. Still she made no progress. The dose was then increased to twenty drops, without much result; but upon again increasing the dose to thirty drops the most immediate improvement resulted. The specific gravity of the urine became higher, the quantity of albumen lessened. The dropsy steadily diminished as the amount of urine increased (from 30 to 45, 50, and eventually to 60 oz.), and the strength and activity soon surprised all her friends, who had given her up as hopelessly lost. The same medicine was continued for three months, and at the end of that time the most careful examination failed to detect albumen or blood-globules in her urine, which was then perfectly transparent, of a clear amber color, and its specific gravity 1023. Every vestige of dropsy was removed, and the catamenia appeared with perfect restoration of health and strength, which has continued up to the present time.

The true physician must rise above prejudice or routine. When satisfied as to his true insight into the nature of the case, and of the suitability of the remedy, he is not to abandon it in haste if no result follows from a small dose, but gradually to increase it till satisfied of having obtained all the efficacy of the medicine.

The physiological action of iodide of potassium is one of similarity to its curative action in coryza, ozæna, catarrh of the Eustachian tubes, of the bronchial mucous membrane, desquamative nephritis. It is that of contrary to the tertiary and secondary syphilis, yet the physician is glad of its help in either case.

Mr. S. for seven weeks suffered much distress from a severe attack of catarrh of the nose, throat, and middle ear, accompanied with soreness of throat, distressing deafness, and sense of thickness and stuffing of the nose and ears. I prescribed four grains of iodide of potassium three times a day. In two days it afforded the most marked relief; in fact, six doses perfectly restored the hearing, to his infinite relief. He left off the medicine, and there was no return of the symptoms —the usual result of a perfect action of "similars." What a contrast in that respect is the following case, illustrating the "contraria contrariis" use of iodide of potassium.

A gentleman, æt. 42, suffered for three months from

a severe ulcerated throat, secondary to an indurated chancre. He was treated by Mr. Gay, and the late Sir B. Brodie, by means of mercurial fumigations to the throat, and moderate doses of mercury internally.

Suffering terrible pain in the throat week after week without any relief, he discontinued their mercurial treatment, and sent for me. I prescribed five grains of iodide of potassium in distilled water three times a day. The relief to pain was immediate, and the ulceration rapidly healed. In three or four days he was at business again. He continued the iodide for ten days, then left it off, supposing himself to be cured. Four days afterwards the throat became as painful as ever; the ulceration reappeared. He resumed the five-grain dose of iodide, and in a few days was again perfectly well. "I accept my condition," said he. "The mercury made me worse and worse for three months; I will take the iodide the instant I feel the relapse." Thus he went on for twelve years—a week of the iodide, a week or ten days without, and so on, never able to leave it off longer than ten days, the palliative action keeping the disease in check, but not curing it permanently, although aided by the use of Turkish baths, careful regulation of the diet, clothing, open air exercise, etc.

What a boon to the patient when a dexterous knowledge of the science and art of medicine enables the doctor to prescribe what cures the disease permanently, and does not require perpetual dosing!

Neuralgia of the Eyes, with Conjunctivitis and Impairment of Sight, cured by Arsenic.—Miss ——, æt.

25, a vigorous, healthy-looking young lady, consulted me in July, 1867. For five years she had suffered from aching pains in the eyeballs, with photophobia, which unfitted her for reading or working. The conjunctiva of both eyes looked red and swollen; pupils natural.

For years she had been under the care of London oculists and physicians with only temporary relief. She had taken iron and quinine in large doses, and used many lotions, including atropia. From the peculiar appearance of the conjunctiva I prescribed arsenic (four drops of Fowler's solution three times a day). The effect was magical. It perfectly cured her in one month, without any local application.

In the healthy human subject the administration of arsenic produces redness of the conjunctiva, watering of the eyes, and photophobia.

It is most important to see that almost *every* fresh discovery in medical *art* sooner or later proves obedient to the rule of law. Dr. John Chapman's interesting application of heat or cold to the spine, in a most singular degree follows the law of "similia similibus curantur." "At a meeting of English physicians in Paris, at the house of Sir Joseph Olliffe, M.D., Physician to the English Embassy, Dr. John Chapman, of London, has given an exposition of his discovery of a new method of treating disease by controlling the circulation of the blood in different parts of the body, through the agency of the nervous system. This he does by cold or heat, or both together, applied along the spine. Having referred to the fact that the arteries

are surrounded by muscular bands, and that these
bands, forming collectively what is called the muscular
coat, contract and dilate at the bidding of nerves ema-
nating from an assemblage of nervous centres, or ganglia, constituting the 'great sympathetic,' he showed
that these ganglia can be so influenced by suitable applications of cold or heat on each side of the spine as to
cause them to effect either the contraction or dilatation
of the arteries which they govern, and that the spinal
cord itself can be influenced in the same way, and can
thus have the circulation of the blood in it, and therefore its functional activity, increased or decreased at
the will of the physician. Fevers of all kinds, including cholera, he treats both by cold and heat—*cold in
the cold stage, heat in the hot;* and affirmed that heat
along the spine will cause the pulse to fall, and will
induce perspiration—abolishing, in fact, the feverish
condition. Spitting of blood and pulmonary hæmorrhage can, he said, be speedily arrested by the proper
application of heat between the shoulderblades. His
own experience on this point was confirmed by that of
Professor Beneke, of Marburg, who, in the *Archiv
für wissenschaftliche Heilkunde*, reports that by adopting Dr. Chapman's method he caused the rapid arrest
of pulmonary hæmorrhage in an obstinate case of long
standing. Dr. Routh said he had tried the method in
a case of profuse menorrhagia; after the double col-
umn hot-water bag had been applied during an hour
the flow ceased."

Feverishness and Fever.—Dr. Chapman says, in the
Introduction to his work on *Diarrhœa and Cholera*,

p. 15: "I have had but slight experience in the treatment of fever, but I anticipate that fevers of all kinds will be most effectually controlled by *cold along the spine in the cold stage* when the bloodvessels are contracted, and heat *in the hot* when they are relaxed."

In a lecture on "Pain" by Mr. Skey, at St. Bartholomew's Hospital, in 1870, he teaches the law of similars most thoroughly and effectively. "The principle I am anxious to insist on as far preferable to any involved in the carron-oil treatment is exhibited in the results of the application of heat to any small burn on the hand, as from a drop of melted scaling-wax. The very smart pain occasioned by this trivial accident is entirely relieved by immersing the hand in hot water, or by holding the hand to the fire for a few minutes. If this be a fact, viz., that by the brief application of an agent promoting pain (for *heat* is not essential) one important element of the injury, that of pain, is quickly relieved, there must be some virtue in the principle involved. And there is a virtue, and a very important one; for I maintain, from many years' experience in the treatment of burns, that not only is the pain far more quickly relieved, but that the cure is hastened in the same proportion.

"Some half a century since this principle of treatment by local stimulants was enunciated to the profession by Dr. Kentish, of Bristol. Its value was at once acknowledged by observing men; and I think I am not mistaken in asserting that the principle was adopted in the majority of the hospitals of the metropolis, if not in all. I know that it was thoroughly appreciated by my own teacher, Mr. Abernethy, who would naturally influence the opinions of a considerable proportion of the profession. The agent employed by Dr. Kentish was spirit of turpentine, which was applied, diluted or otherwise, over the affected surface. The application was accompanied by an increase of temporary pain, which, however, passed off in the course of a few hours, and thus improved the condition of the patient. The amount of pain was in relation with the extent and severity of each injury.

" I wish to recommend to your recollection the employment of a remedy on the same principle I have for many years resorted to both in St. Bartholomew's Hospital and elsewhere, viz., a solution of nitrate of silver in a proportionate strength to the extent and severity of the burn. I have used the solution in the strength of from five to twelve or more grains to the ounce of water. The lotion would, of course, be modified by the age of the person—five grains, or about five, sufficing for a child. If the whole surface be freely bathed with the solution, and entirely covered up in cotton-wool, and a moderate opiate be administered in a glass of brandy and water in strength proportioned to the age and habits of the patient, with the object of counteracting the sense of chilliness that will otherwise necessarily follow in all these cases, I think you will find you have made a good start in the future management of your case. In all cases, whether of burn or scald of the external skin, I say resort to local stimulants. The soft and soothing system, I believe, answers no useful purpose whatever beyond that of excluding air, if that be, as supposed, a great desideratum.

"The theory of the excellent results of the treatment of burns by provocatives, or remedies that provoke physical pain, is not very clear. It would appear that relief invariably follows a temporary increase of pain; but one is inclined to ask whether the benefit consists in the actual presence of pain, and how far the same agency—whether of fire, hot water, turpentine, or the nitrate of silver lotion—would be equally beneficial when the subject of the injury was placed under the influence of chloroform. This question I must refer to others more fortunate than I in having at their command a larger field of inquiry than now falls to my lot. My advice to you is to abjure carron oil and all demulcents, and to adopt the treatment of burns and scalds by local stimuli."*

* Mr. Skey, Lancet, August 27th, 1870.

CHAPTER IX.

ARS MEDICA.

In the present age of specialists it is needful for the consulting physician to train his hand as well as his brain and eyes. Without undervaluing the genius and skill of many that are called specialists, it is far better for the patient, in many cases, to be treated by the general physician not only for the health, but also for the local disease. The doctor who has most science should not have the less art, although Trousseau said in one of his lectures, " Let us have less science, but more art." The loss of one could ill supplement the other.

It is often an advantage to the patient to be kept from the hands of the specialist—now often only a " bookmaker," without the adroitness that constitutes the perfect helper to suffering humanity.

Miss ——, æt. 23, suffered for a year from constant nausea and vomiting, which resisted all treatment. Tracing back the cause, it appeared that the day the sickness first came on she had a fall in stepping out of a carriage. As all ordinary means had failed to cure, I examined the uterus, and found decided retroflexion. Having replaced the uterus, I inserted the air-ball pessary. The next day nausea and vomiting perfectly ceased. At once she was lifted out of a life of suffering and invalidism into health and activity.

Miss ——, æt. 32, for upwards of three years suffered from total inability to walk, with distressing pain at the back of the head and vertex. For a year she was confined to the couch, so as to have the influence of "perfect rest," without any relief. Then the doctor tried to persuade her that she was better, and urged walking, which much aggravated the congestive headache. She then came to London, and was treated for some time by a well-known specialist physician. He detected retroversion, lifted up the displaced womb, *and left it so.* For three or four days she could walk perfectly, but gradually all the old misery and distress returned. Thus he went on treating her for six or eight months, lifting up the womb every three or four weeks, each time giving her a few days' relief. Discouraged with this temporary patching up, she went to another, a well-known surgeon. He attempted to replace the womb by means of the uterine sound, but gave her such agonizing pain that she went straight from his house and sent for me. I found the retroverted fundus wedged in under the promontory of the sacrum. Administering chloroform just enough to dull sensation, I replaced the womb according to the plan of my friend, Marion Sims, inserted a Hodge's * pessary with a long

---

* Uterine therapeutics owe much to America. Dr. Hodge, of Philadelphia, seems to be the first who conceived that in cases of displacement of the uterus, the means of support should take the exact shape of the pelvis ; and in place of taking a rigid standpoint, should lie floating in the moisture of the vaginal

curve, and kept her on the face in bed for twenty-four hours. The result was all that could be desired. She went back to the country perfectly well in a few days; could walk and stand, and for two years remained free from headache.

She required no attention of any sort for eighteen months, then only that the vulcanite of the pessary softened and lost its curve. One visit set it to rights, and she remains active and well.

Miss ——, æt. 26, a lady of highly nervous organization, but most active disposition, suddenly became unable to walk or stand. She was attended by the family doctor for a long time. He assured her father and mother that "it was all hysteria." Unable to cure her, he summoned a London accoucheur physician to a consultation, who examined the womb, and agreed with the family doctor, saying "she could walk if she wished and tried." The poor lady knew he was wrong. The one thing her whole nature craved for was to get about amongst the sick poor of her father's parish. She knew also that the two doctors' opinions had made her parents wretched. They loved her deeply, and knew what her life had been to many a weary one. Now to see her laid aside from all service, and from self-will, according to the London doctor's opinion!* She bore all with

walls, and thus take on a lever action by the inclination of the upper segment.

Hodge's pessary, variously modified, proves itself the most perfect of all mechanical arrangements in remedying retroflexion of the uterus.

* Alas! it was the very same specialist who had proved of

patience, helplessly confined to her bed for many months. A friend who knew her former life of active usefulness sent me to see her. On examination I found the fundus uteri indurated, much enlarged, retroflexed, and wedged into the hollow of the sacrum. I explained to the anxious mother that for all the so-called hysteria there was a tangible physical cause, the removal of which would enable her to walk. It was a difficult case; required the full effects of chloroform to relax all muscular exertion. Then with ease I lifted up and replaced the uterus, and inserted a Hodge's pessary. In a few days the congested, indurated womb had become soft and reduced in size. She could walk and stand as well as ever, and before the end of the week was out visiting amongst the poor, as of old. For three years she continued well; then, from overexertion, relapse occurred, which a little adroitness soon set right. The precious result of the *ars medica* was a great boon to the aged father, beholding the simple, natural life at once restored, and his old faith in his child again realized.

Lady ——, æt. 43, consulted me in 1870. For many years she suffered from a fibroid tumor of the uterus, causing backache and inability to walk. From time to time she had consulted most of the leading

---

such little use to the case previously mentioned. If argument was needed to show the ill effect of specialists it is to be found in their frequent unskilfulness and carelessness. Success in getting practice seems to change many of them into mere routinists, riding their one hobby, taking things easy, and too often ceasing to afford real help.

specialists in London, Vienna, Berlin, Edinburgh.
She got no help from any one except from the late Mr.
Baker Brown, who afforded her nearly two years' relief
by an operation. After two years she became as bad
as ever, and consulted me. I found the fibroid tumor
the size of a billiard-ball, low down in the pelvis, fill-
ing up the hollow of the sacrum, and much impeding
defecation. With much patience and perseverance I
lifted up the tumor, and got most, if not all, above
the brim of the pelvis. Before it fell back to its old
place, keeping her lying in the prone position, I fitted
in the largest size Hodge's pessary, so as to push up
the vagina and make it tense. By keeping her much
in the prone position for some days, careful attention
to softening the evacuations from the bowels to prevent
straining, much to her and my surprise, the tumor kept
up. She could walk without the slightest pain or difficulty. The pessary was kept in for two years, and
then withdrawn. There was no recurrence of the
symptoms; she has remained perfectly well ever since.
Here art used means very effectual, yet simple, in con-
tradistinction to Baker Brown's severe cutting operation.

The unpretending simple-looking uterine sponge-
tent has led to the exploration and cure of many cases
of uterine disease that before its use were considered
among the incurable cases, too often confounded with
cancer and given up in despair, till the patient died of
hæmorrhage or exhaustion.

In 186–, a lady, aged 44, consulted me for frequent
and profuse loss at the catamenial periods, which, from

the ordinary duration of five or six days increased to
ten days, causing pallor, anæmia, exhaustion, and inability to walk.   After a most careful examination by
the touch and by the speculum, I could detect no cause
for this prostrating hæmorrhage, which no treatment
seemed to cure.   After a few months she went to
another doctor with the same result, then to a third—
all to no use.   About two years after she first consulted
me, I was summoned to see her.   She thought herself dying, had lain on the bed for six weeks, fainting
on the least exertion, from constant flooding.   She
looked deadly pale, was nearly pulseless, and could
scarcely speak.   Her husband thought life was fast
ebbing.   Upon examining her, I detected a small
fibroid tumor projecting through the os uteri, which
was large, soft, and patulous.   Two years before it
was small and perfectly natural.   To remove the little
growth by the scissors seemed to lift her at once into
health.   In a fortnight she was able to get out and
walk, rapidly regained color and strength, and has remained perfectly well ever since.   This case proved a
most instructive lesson, and taught me what nature had
been doing in the two years.   Not long afterwards, an
unmarried lady, aged 51, sent for me.   For ten or
eleven years she had been flooding at the monthly
periods, and had been under treatment for most of that
time without much relief.   She said, " I have been
flooding for years, but I feel I cannot survive another
attack like the last, which caused such deathlike and
prolonged fainting that I want to know can anything
be done to prevent the loss?"   I examined her most

carefully by the finger and the speculum. The os
uteri looked small, soft, natural, no sign of ulceration.
The body of the womb was not enlarged, no hardness,
no displacement. I explained to her that although
ordinary examination could not discover the cause, yet
I had sufficient grounds for the suspicion of the existence of a tumor inside the upper part of the womb, and
that the only mode of detection was by the use of the
sponge-tent to open up the cavity of the womb. In a
few days she took rooms in London. With the help
of a friend the cervical canal was fully expanded by
sponge-tents, then — under chloroform — the fundus
uteri was explored by the finger, and a small fibroid
tumor discovered attached to its upper part. This was
grasped by the long vulsella forceps, and removed by
the scissors. She recovered from the chloroform to learn
that the cause of all her sufferings had been removed,
and made an excellent recovery. The next monthly
period came on very moderately, and at the right time.
The floodings never returned, and her health became
perfectly restored. She is still alive and well.

Mrs. B., aged 28, consulted me in 1868, suffering
from extreme depression and melancholy, because of
the disappointment of having no child, although four
years married. She was the more unhappy because a
London physician-accoucheur had used sponge-tents
to dilate the uterine canal without any result. On
examination, I found the os uteri large and soft, but
the upper part of the cervical canal narrow and contracted. On account of the previous failure, I took
extra care with the use of sponge-tents; passed the
third, a very long one, right through the internal os.

This brought on sharp pain for twelve hours, but the result was most successful. Two months afterwards she conceived, and went safely through to her confinement at the full time.

The more perfect in science the physician, the more adroit should he be in art.

Mr. ——, æt 36, a burly-looking gentleman farmer, from the neighborhood of Chelmsford, came into my consulting-room on crutches, without which he had been unable to get about for upwards of a year. His legs hung flaccid, as if paralyzed; yet every essential sign of disease of brain or spine was absent. Searching for the cause, I discovered a chronic gleet that had existed for eight years, and a stricture so tight that a No. 1 bougie could with difficulty be passed. He took lodgings in London. Beginning with No. 1, in the course of six weeks I succeeded in passing No. 8. As the stricture was cured, the gleet ceased of itself, and the power of walking returned perfectly. After six weeks, he went back to Chelmsford, to the surprise of all his friends, able to walk without the crutches.

The Bishop of ——, returned from his post on the coast of Africa, for the second time invalided for debility caused by loss of blood from piles, which had existed for four years. He had been treated by the colonial surgeon, afterwards by two surgeons in London and a physician at Brighton; but the cause was not discovered till he came to me. After the action of the bowels, I examined, and found a large villous pile, about an inch up, exuding blood profusely. Wiping this with a wet sponge, I touched the sur-

face with the strongest nitric acid. This caused very
little pain, and after three applications he was perfectly cured, had no return of bleeding, recovered
strength, and went back to his bishopric. Even the
relaxing climate of the West Coast of Africa did not
cause a return of the bleeding.

Acute Glaucoma, Iridectomy ; cure.—Mrs. ——, the
wife of a clergyman living near Barnet. She had
been treated most vigorously for six weeks by two
local doctors, for what they called "acute ophthalmia."
Leeches, blisters, mercury—all were used freely without relief. I found her in agonizing pain, aggravated
by the slightest trace of light ; eyeballs hard as mar-
bles, pupils dilated. Her distress was aggravated by
the knowledge that her father had precisely such an
attack at her age—about 34—which resulted in total
blindness. To the surprise of the patient and her
husband, I said, "It is not a physician you want, but
an ophthalmic surgeon." I explained the nature of
the case (acute glaucoma), told them it was not yet
too late for an operation of iridectomy, sent a mes-
senger at once with a note to Mr. George Critchett,
and retired from the case. He came down early the
next morning, performed the operation, which perfectly succeeded; at once relieved the tension and
pain that six weeks' strong drugging had failed to do.
The sight became gradually restored. Her own father,
a retired physician, still living, was rejoiced to find
that Von Graafe's great discovery of the cure of glaucoma, saved his child from the blindness which followed his own case.

In many a pure surgical case, the best thing for the physician is promptly to withdraw and summon the pure surgeon; yet the case is not infrequent where the surgeon's art must be pushed aside by the physician's skill.

Mrs. ——, a strong, healthy-looking lady, æt. 26, consulted me for a distressing pain and irritation in the uterus and vagina, which had made her existence miserable for three years, during which she had been under most skilful treatment; for one year under Dr. Marion Sims, at Paris, who operated on her severely although unsuccessfully. The vagina was healthy-looking, no signs of vaginismus; the uterine neck slightly congested, and the os red-looking, although not ulcerated. No treatment seemed to have relieved her, so that she was kept in a state of frenzy and excitement. Observing some little patches on the os uteri like the spots on the tongue in psoriasis of that organ, I prescribed five drops of Fowler's solution of arsenic three times a day. This proved a cure for all her misery. After two or three weeks' use of it, large spots of psoriasis came out on her wrists and forearms, and all the uterine distress passed away permanently. After the arsenic had thrown out the psoriasis on her wrists, her father noticed it, and showed her the same on his forearm, which had existed for twenty-five years. This lady had gone through prolonged and painful surgical treatment at the hands of the most experienced uterine surgeons for this medical disease, which obeyed the touch of law, and was cured by a few weeks' specific medical treat-

ment after three years of unsuccessful surgical treatment.

Mr. A., æt. 41, nervous, sanguine temperament, became affected with agonizing pain in the back, shooting
into the lower extremities, for which his spine was blis-
tered by a London physician without any benefit.
After suffering thus for five or six weeks, these parox-
ysms of pain suddenly ceased, and severe neuralgic
headache set in. This continued off and on for some
months, and then ceased; but was soon followed by most
distressing spasms and gnawing pain at the pit of the
stomach, with sudden twitchings in the limbs, which
kept him, off and on for six months, in a state of incessant nervous agitation and distress. He consulted
many of the most distinguished London physicians,
including Dr. Brown-Séquard, with only occasional
palliative relief.

Again and again the same distressing, agonizing attacks came on. He went into a hydropathic establishment at Malvern for six weeks, and got much worse
under a lowering regimen of farinaceous food and very
little or no meat. In an agony of despair, his dis-
tracted wife telegraphed for me to visit him at Malvern.
After a day of good feeding, and a liberal use of brandy
and water, I removed him to his own house, near London, where for many weeks he was fed upon abundance
of fresh meat and a liberal supply of port wine.

Under this generous regimen the Malvern doctors'
bugbear, " the inflammation of the mucous membrane,"
vanished, the patient recovered strength, and the ab-

dominal neuralgia became suspended.   After three or
four months, the attack of neuralgic pain in the stomach came on again.   He then laid aside all medicine,
and derived much benefit from horse-riding.   After
some time he got as bad as ever.   I prescribed cod-
liver oil and the use of continuous-current galvanism,
with only temporary benefit.

Examining the urine I found many spermatozoa.
Searching for the cause of this, I discovered a well-
marked fissure in the rectum, where he had at times
much burning pain.   I touched the bottom of the
fissure with strong nitric acid, and in less than five
minutes all his neuralgic pain ceased.   The good effect
lasted for some days.   The application was repeated
three or four times, at a week's interval.   The same in-
stantaneous relief followed each time, but, as it proved
only temporary, he submitted to the knife; free divi-
sion of the fissure through the sphincter perfectly cured
him.

This case is a well-marked illustration that even in
diseases of internal organs the exact cause must be
searched for.   Till that is touched skilfully, there is
no real cure, which often rewards the most dexterous
searcher who possesses more art but not less science.

For the improvement of the "art of medicine," the
scientific physician has to follow the line of progress
opened up for him by the surgeon, especially in the
careful elaboration and practical management of details bearing upon treatment.   Of all the lessons which
surgical art has yet given to medicine, the antiseptic

treatment by Professor Lister* stands foremost in results. In the expressive words of Dr. Parkes,† "Bacteria, infinitesimally small yet infinitely active, penetrate from without by the surface of wounds, or at times by the intestinal surface. These small cells pass into the bloodvessels, in which they live and multiply, probably blocking up the channel. Others are carried by the living cells to distant parts, to cause diseases that indicate the need of antiseptic medicine as well as of antiseptic surgery."

That the formation of bacteria is invariably prevented in the pus of wounds treated antiseptically is still *sub judice*. Dr. Bastian has made himself famous by opposing Pasteur, Lister, and Tyndall; yet no scientific mind accepts Dr. Bastian's doctrine.

What science in reality needs to know is if the pus

---

* In the domain of surgery, Professor Lister had demonstrated in his antiseptic treatment that the putrefaction of wounds was to be averted by the destruction of bacteria. Passing from surgery to the domain of medicine, he said the conviction was spreading and growing daily in strength, that reproductive parasitic life was at the root of epidemic disease—that living ferments finding lodgment in the body increased there and multiplied, directly ruining the tissue on which they subsisted, or destroying life indirectly by the generation of poisonous compounds within the body. This conclusion, which came to us with a presumption almost amounting to demonstration, had been clinched by the fact that virulently infective diseases had been discovered with which living organisms were as closely and as indissolubly connected as the growth of torula was with the fermentation of beer.—The Germ Theory of Disease by Professor Tyndall.

† Lancet, August 9th, 1873.

of wounds treated without the antiseptic precautions by perfect cleanliness and excluding of the open air, differs essentially from the pus flowing—often freely—from under the elaborate antiseptic dressing.

If both alike contain bacteria, the antiseptic theory falls to the ground, yet the lesson of elaborate care and infrequent dressing of wounds remains.

Professor Lister's gauze looks clumsy, and does not exclude air so well as cotton-wool, which absorbs the carbolic mixture quite as freely as the gauze, and covers the wound much more accurately.

CHAPTER X.

OBSTACLES TO THE ACTION OF MEDICINE.

THE study of heart diseases is one of the most interesting and complex of all studies. Here it is that a sound knowledge of chemical and mechanical laws is essential to successful treatment, as well as an intimate acquaintance with the laws of the nervous system, which uses and co-ordinates the physical forces. The dropsy from heart disease increases more slowly than the dropsy caused by disease of kidneys. The latter is much relieved by vapor, or Turkish, or hot baths, which generally aggravate the dropsy from heart disease. Dropsy from disease of kidneys can be cured without purgatives, but dropsy from heart disease, with constipation, finds no relief from any treatment till the constipation is relieved, when the specific heart medicine acts like a charm on the dropsy. Dropsy from heart disease is more often seen in the serous membranes. It usually shows first on the left side, whilst œdema from obstruction of liver almost invariably commences on the right side. Dropsy caused by disease of kidneys affects both sides much alike.

Obstruction from Ossification, causing Permanent Patency of the Mitral Valve; Ascites.—Miss C., æt. 36, suffered from gradually increasing dyspnœa, especially in ascending. Œdema gradually came on. Not getting relief in the country, she came to London. I found her unable to lie down from a hacking, dry cough, dulness on percussion all over the base of the left lung, feeble respiratory murmur with moist crepitation. The abdomen much distended, with evident fluctuation. Pulse 110. Bowels regular. Urine scanty, 16 oz. in twenty-four hours. Specific gravity 1020, containing a copious deposit of lithate of ammonia, non-albuminous.

I prescribed infusion of digitalis, half an ounce three times a day. The second day after taking it, the urine increased from one to four pints in the twenty-four hours, and four days afterwards to six pints; the dropsy speedily decreased, and in about a fortnight she was able to lie flat in bed without cough. The percussion became quite clear all over the base of the left lung, and she could take moderate exercise without any difficulty of breathing. She returned to Reading, and remained quite well for nearly half a year; then the dropsy gradually returned. She came up to London again, but the state of the heart was evidently much worse. The most urgent orthopnœa soon came on. The digitalis was given again, but in vain, as the dropsy increased, and after a few weeks' hard struggle she died. Post-mortem examination showed the mitral valve converted into a perfect ring of bone.

Miss K. S., æt. 6, a sensitive, nervous child, got a sudden shock early in 1869 from the father unexpectedly going to California, fretted much for many months, and in June became prostrated, unable to walk. Swelling of the legs came on, gradually followed by ascites and oedema of the lungs. She had been under the care of a local doctor and of a London physician for six or eight weeks. The dropsy increasing, I was called to see her, found her limbs and body enormously swollen, dulness at the base of the right lung, with absence of respiratory murmur. Pulse 132, feeble, loud systolic murmur over the region of the mitral valve. The area of cardiac dulness much increased. Urine, only ten ounces in twenty-four hours, pale, low specific gravity 1010, non-albuminous. Bowels rather loose.

I prescribed digitalis—two teaspoonfuls of the infusion every four hours, and a generous diet, with a glass of champagne twice a day. Gradually the quantity of urine increased, the dropsy lessened, and in a few weeks she was perfectly cured.

The case is interesting as a clinical fact—perfect restoration to health from the use of a single remedy, without adjuncts, beyond good food and wine.

About two years afterwards a relapse occurred, the heart's action became weaker, the dropsy slowly returned as badly as ever. The same remedy, the infusion of digitalis, was again carefully administered for many weeks, but without result. Even when the dose was pushed to a tablespoonful three times a day still there was no diminution of the dropsy, no improvement in the heart's action, and no increase of urine. I then prescribed in addition to the digitalis half an ounce of sulphate of magnesia in a wine-glass of water, each morning. In a few days the quantity of urine increased, and the dropsy was again perfectly cured, the heart's action improving, and she got up out of bed where she had lain for eight weeks. By degrees she recovered strength, and got about as well as ever, and for a period of nearly three years remained, to all appearances, well—still with all the signs of cardiac enlargement and mitral dilatation.

Again the dropsy slowly returned, the abdomen became so large and distended that she lay in bed for nearly three months unable to stir, even to move herself, without help. Digitalis was again given, the infusion first, afterwards changed to the tincture, in eight-minim doses. No effect was produced on the dropsy. Again help of the purgative was added, yet no result whatever towards cure. I feared that the end of life was slowly coming on. Watching the utter prostration of muscular power, I omitted the purgative and prescribed six drops of the pure tincture of nux vomica twice a day before meals, and continued the infusion of digitalis, a dessertspoonful three times a day a couple of hours after meals. The nux vomica acted like a charm. At once the former effects of the digitalis showed itself, the quantity of urine rapidly increased, the dropsy lessened, the muscular power returned. In two or three days she sat up in bed and began to exert herself. In a fortnight or three weeks she was up and as full of play as ever. Since then she has kept well, with occasional relapses, which three or four days' use of the nux vomica and digitalis soon rights.

Mr. ——, æt. 62, a thin, sallow-looking city gentleman, for many years subject to weak action of the heart, was suddenly seized at his warehouse with breath-

lessness, palpitation, and inability to walk. Gradually
dropsy came on. He was treated for nearly two months
by a well-known West-end physician. The case was
so urgent that for several weeks this gentleman slept
in the patient's house. The dropsy steadily increased,
till the patient's abdomen and legs became enormously
swollen, so much so that he lay on his back unable to
move from side to side for nearly a fortnight. The
close attention of his medical friend having proved useless to the patient, as a last resource, when life seemed
coming near its close, he sent for Dr. Hewan, who
summoned me to a consultation.

The former medical attendant retired from the case,
leaving eleven different medicines on the table, all in use,
each for some symptom of the disease; one for the palpitation, one for the dropsy, another for the bowels, a
fourth for the breathing, and so on; directions written
out for each of the eleven medicines, with two nurses to
superintend their administration. The patient lay like
a log in bed, all the cellular tissue of the body, even to
the eyelids and forehead, œdematous, swollen; the peri-
toneum distended with fluid. The heart's action feeble,
muffled with a soft systolic " bruit," audible over the
region of the mitral valve. The area of dulness over
the region of the heart much increased. Universal
crepitation over the base of both lungs. The urine
scanty, dark-colored, free from albumen; bowels costive.

We prescribed infusion of digitalis, half an ounce
three times a day, without any sensible relief. The
dose was increased to one ounce, yet no effect. Afterwards ten-drop doses of the tincture of digitalis were
given; still no increase of urine, no relief to the dropsy

or the dyspnœa.   Beginning to lose heart, Dr. Hewan
said at our next consultation, "We must give up the
digitalis."   "No," was my reply; "but we must remove the obstacles to its action."   Accordingly, a brisk
mercurial purgative was prescribed at bedtime, and the
digitalis continued, a tablespoonful three times a day.

Twenty-four hours after the purgative, the true
action of the digitalis showed itself in the free secretion
of urine, which for many weeks had been scanty,
averaging 20 ounces in the twenty-four hours.   Within two days it increased to 50 ounces—on the third day
to 60 ounces.   Before the end of the week it reached
100 ounces.   It was continued in tablespoonful doses
for a week, then reduced to a dessert-spoonful, and
after a few days to a teaspoonful; yet upwards of 100
ounces of urine continued to flow daily for three weeks.
Then the quantity gradually decreased to 50 ounces.
The dropsy slowly vanished, breathing became easy,
and in a month, to the amazement of a very numerous
circle of friends, the patient got about, apparently quite
well.   He lived for nearly three years.   Eventually,
dilatation of the heart increased, and the dropsy came on
again.   With the increase of organic disease, there was
less response to treatment, and he died, suffocated with
dropsy into the pericardium and pleura.

In this case the digitalis, unaided, had no curative
action.   It was given in small doses, in large doses,
in tincture, fluid extract, and fresh-made infusion (from
several chemists, too).   The infusion was also applied
externally as a compress over the kidneys and abdomen; yet, although producing depression of pulse,

loss of appetite and strength, it was about being laid aside altogether as useless, when the brisk action of the purgative relieved the obstructed portal circulation, like delicate clockwork kept from going by the mainspring being weighed down. The obstacle being removed, then the digitalis acted like a charm, gradually increasing the urine from 20 ounces to 100 ounces, carrying off the dropsy to its last vestige. The old man was moved from his warehouse, where he was first seized, to his house in the country, and lived for three years a life of comparative comfort.

To remove the obstacles which oppose recovery, and change the unfavorable conditions into favorable, affords the most admirable field for the exercise of skill on the part of the doctor.

In acute bronchitis, giving the direct specific, he finds how much it helps recovery to moisten the air of the room—to keep the temperature equable day and night, to interdict moving or talking, give nutritious unstimulating diet in rather moderate quantities, encourage free secretions of the skin, of the kidneys, and of the bowels; thus he brings all indirect means to help the direct effect of the specific; then, indeed, the physician becomes the friend of the sick man, in every way doing good and held back from doing mischief by the knowledge of laws reigning over the processes of health and disease.

The following was a case of impending suffocation from bronchitis relieved by the use of steam:

Mrs. A., æt. 62, living in Gower Street, of feeble constitution, had been subject for many years to asthma

14

and palpitation. From exposure to cold east winds in March, 1860, she was seized with acute bronchitis of both sides. I found her with a weak fluttering pulse, 125; hot, dry skin; distressing, dry cough, with very scanty viscid expectoration, unable to lie down or to sleep day or night from the dyspnœa and difficulty of expectoration. She was treated vigorously, mustard poultices frequently applied, a large fire kept up day and night, with wet sheets all round the fires. Beef tea, brandy and water, administered freely; the bowels well emptied by stimulating injections. She continued in the same state of suffering for four days without relief. When life seemed ebbing, I sent for a portable vapor-bath kettle, with a tin spout ten feet long, and set it furiously boiling into the room, which in a few hours it filled with a delicious soft vapor. The effect was marvellous, the old lady began to cough up quantities of thick expectoration, consciousness returned, and she recovered from the semi-comatose state of carbonized blood-poisoning. She lived for two or three years, and several times before her death derived signal relief in attacks of bronchitis from the use of steam in the room.

CHAPTER XI.

THE LAW OF COUNTER-IRRITATION.

THE laws of counter-irritation are clear and decided; whether we incline to Dr. Risden Bennett's theory of depletion, or to Dr. Anstie's of stimulation, the facts are true. In the words of Hippocrates, "a stronger pain can mask a weaker."

"The idea of counter-irritation is to supersede one morbid action by another."*

If two sets of capillaries are in intimate connection, we may relieve one by drawing blood from the other. A severe superficial irritation relieves the deeper organ when its function is embarrassed with acute inflammation.

Whether we regard the part irritated and the organ to be acted upon as in communication through the nervous system or the vascular, or through the cellular tissue, the primary law of counter-irritation is "similia similibus."

The best results from counter-irritation are as the application follows that law. The most searching and curative application is *near the organ affected*, yet a little

---

* Dr. Dickinson, The Practitioner, vol. iii, p. 99.

removed from it; or over another organ whose function or sympathy is allied, as over the breasts to influence the ovaries and uterus, or *vice versa.*

Counter-irritation acts best when the organ to be acted upon is in an excited state akin to itself, such as asthma, or bronchitis, or of painful diseases like pleurisy or pericarditis. Blisters in neuralgia are most effectual on the posterior roots of the nerves, *i. e.* the painful application over the most painful or sensitive spot.*

As long as the organ or function is in a state of irritation it derives help from counter-irritation, but in its ordinary passive state it does not prove susceptible even to most powerful counter-irritation.

"Milder counter-irritants in the early stages, stronger in the later stage of inflammation to promote absorption of the products thereof.

"In chronic cases of disease which require a good deal of stimulation, a blister has a more marked effect than a mustard poultice, a pustular eruption than a blister, and an issue or a seton than a pustular eruption." †

"Injection of hydrocele by iodine to excite a subacute inflammation for the sake of its resulting curative adhesion, in order to displace a chronic inflammation secreting serum of low type organization. The path of disease becomes the channel of therapeutic influence. Burns, especially of the abdominal integuments, induce ulceration of the duodenum, a hint for the therapeutic

---

* Dr. Anstie, The Practitioner, vol. iv, p. 165.
† Dr. Ross, The Practitioner, vol. iv, p. 83.

employment of vesication of the epigastrium in the treatment of duodenal or pyloric disease."*

The more akin to the disease is the therapeutic counter-irritation the more permanent the relief. Eczema of the skin in children—a natural counter-irritation, frequently relieves catarrh of the bronchial mucous membrane. The latter often becomes aggravated on the subsidence of the former.

Counter-irritation at a distance also has an excellent effect, as the use of hot mustard foot-baths in congestive headache, in brain-irritation, or acute mania; mustard poultices at the back of the neck in painful states of the brain, as severe neuralgia or acute headache at vertex; hot mustard arm-bath in restlessness from heart disease, or asthma, or spinal irritation.

Certain organs have most intimate sympathies with other organs, as proved by the effect of a leech or two to the anus, or of a dose of aloes in vascular fulness of the brain.

The use of counter-irritation is the more beneficial the more it is prescribed under the reign of law of similars or of contraries. In painful conditions the effect of mustard is to excite a fresh condition of pain that excludes or overpowers the natural pain. If the latter be superficial, the application of mustard will suffice; if deepseated, it is more under the control of the more powerful agent, such as iodine, whose action is more profound and searching.

The first stage of blistering is similar to the condition

---

* Dr. Risden Bennett, The Practitioner, vol. ii, p. 333.

of recent inflammation of serous-membrane, which it often arrests if applied before actual effusion has occurred. If applied early, the tendency to effusion may be arrested, and with it the resulting adhesion of the pleura, which more or less impedes free respiration through the rest of life.

The final action of the blister is similar to the last stage of the effusion. When effusion into the pericardium has occurred, free diuresis gives more relief than any other treatment, exuding of fluid through the kidneys carrying off the exudation into the serous sac.

When counter-irritation is applied according to the relationship of similarity, i. e., near to, but not upon a painful part, the effect is quickly beneficial, and the diseased action often does not recur. When the application is discontinued—in the same manner as when a medicine's activity in relationship of similar is omitted —the disease does not return.

A seton or issue at the back of the neck is unlike the diseased process in epilepsy. Accordingly it requires to be kept up indefinitely, as directly the issue is allowed to heal the fits return; exactly as the use of bromide of potassium cannot be discontinued without relapse.

A gentleman on the Stock Exchange suffered for three years from distressing headache; constant dull aching in the forehead and vertex. After the unavailing use of much treatment—medicinal, dietetic, hydropathic—he got immediate relief from a small blister on the left arm. For the past five years he has kept free from headache, as long as he keeps the blister

going, once in fourteen days.   If allowed perfectly to
dry up, the distress in the head returns.

Mr. ——, æt. 36, of a highly nervous temperament,
suffered from nervous distress, with sinking at epigastrium, faintness, sudden attacks of spasms in the stomach.   He remained in a most distressing condition for
nearly two years, at times better, but never quite well,
till a carbuncle appeared on the back of his neck, when
all the nervous symptoms perfectly disappeared; but
directly the carbuncle healed they returned as badly
as ever.   A few months afterwards another carbuncle
appeared on his shoulder, with the same relief to his
nervous distress.   Before it healed I inserted a pea
into the base of the carbuncle, thus converting it into
a natural issue.   This perfectly and permanently cured
his old disease.   The issue was kept open for two years.
At the end of a year half a pea was used; six months
afterwards the size was reduced to quarter of a pea.
Thus very gradually allowed to heal, the old symptoms did not return.

Apropos of issues, about the same time I attended a
gentleman in consumption for whom a well-known
chest doctor had prescribed an issue under the clavicle.
The effect was, in the words of the patient, " to cause
the loss of six pounds of flesh in one week, which was
never regained."   The issue that was natural proved
permanently curative; the issue non-natural proved
most mischievous.

CHAPTER XII.

GALVANISM AND ELECTRO-MAGNETISM.

DUCHESNE, in Paris, was one of the first to lay the foundation of a science of electro-therapeutics. Although his labors were chiefly with the induced or galvano-magnetic current, yet they were very fruitful in results, especially in teaching the importance of localizing the applications.

A more fruitful field of galvano-therapeutics was opened up by the use of the continuous or constant current in Germany by Remak.

Many cases of neuralgia and of diseases of the central nervous system are cured or relieved by the use of the constant galvanic current, upon which the electro-magnetic has no effect but a mischievous one, disturbing and aggravating what the constant current cures or relieves,

The action of galvanism or the continuous current has a much greater analogy than the Faradic or electro-magnetic to the healthy functions of the brain, the spine, liver, kidneys, and other organs. The continuous current is subtle, penetrating, all-pervading, gentle in its action, whilst the magneto-electric is high tension, dashing off upon the surface, unlike the low-tension currents of the nerves. Viewed as elements of a battery, the cells and fibres of the nervous centres are analogous to a galvanic battery of very low tension, composed of countless elements of infinitesimal size— hence the greater efficacy of the continuous current or the galvanic in diseases of the nervous centres, of the liver, and other internal organs.

In disease of internal organs—brain, spine, liver, stomach, intestines, kidneys—the galvanic current is indeed a most valuable aid to treatment.

As yet the application of galvanism to disease of the brain has not borne much fruit, perhaps owing to the imperfection of its mode of application. What seems indicated is a continous current of a number of extremely small cells.

Pulvermacher's chains, to a slight degree, and very imperfectly, meet this need, but there is such an inherent want of constancy and of accuracy that leaves much to be desired for the instrument-maker's ingenuity.

Mrs. P., suffering from deficient action of the liver and of the mucous membrane of the duodenum, passing inspissated bile with temporary jaundice, used the electro-magnetic, or induced current battery, with slight benefit. On changing to the use of Stohrer's 20-cell continuous, she derived great benefit, especially as to the amount of pain, the character of the secretions, and the frequency of the attacks.*

---

* " Professor Burdon Sanderson read his paper on ' Electrical Phenonena which accompany the Contraction of the Leaf of Venus's Flytrap.' He said that in certain plants an irritability was shown which, whether mechanical, chemical, or electrical, was very similar to that which occurred in animals. The obser-

Mrs. M. for three years suffered from jaundice, caused by obstruction of gall-ducts. She derived a little help from the continuous current perseveringly used for many months, but was cured of the jaundice by a few weeks' use of the induced current; one electrode into the rectum, the other pressed tightly over the region of the gall-bladder.

---

vation he would bring before them went far to prove that the electrical action which went on in muscle and nerve occurred also in plants. If we took a portion of living nerve and connected it at both ends by means of a galvanic chain passing through a galvanometer we could prove that the current of electricity set in a constant direction, but whenever the nerve was brought into action the galvanic current immediately ceased; the moment the nerve was irritated, the muscle contracted. The observation he had to make was that a similar phenomenon occurred when the flower commonly called 'Venus's Flytrap,' was treated in a similar manner. This flower, as was well known, had teeth, which under certain circumstances—as when the hairs of the leaf were touched by a fly—immediately closed upon each other and inclosed it. Suppose that one end of the electrode were attached to the end of the petiole nearest the flower leaf, and the other end connected with the part most distant from the leaf, an electrical action set in exactly corresponding to that of the nerve. Let a fly touch the leaf while the current was passing, and the needle of the galvanometer immediately swung back to zero, corresponding again to the nerve action. Vegetable physiologists had very much neglected this branch of inquiry, although as regards animal investigations they were so perfect as to make a new science, under the name of 'Animal Galvanism.' The President (Professor Rutherford) said it had been held by Professor Hermann that electric currents were not produced in living tissues, but the fact now mentioned conclusively showed that electricity was generated in the leaf of the plant without the leaf being destroyed, and it completely settled the question."—The Science of Animal Galvanism, Dr. Burdon Sanderson.

In the first case the continuous current deeply modified the function of the liver, in the second the induced or Faradic powerfully stimulated the ducts and muscular structure of the small intestine.

Neuralgia of the Fifth.—Mrs. —— suffered distressing pain in the face and upper jaw day and night for some weeks; the application of fourteen cells of Stohrer's continuous current, with one electrode over the seat of pain, the other at back of neck, gave no relief; but on putting both electrodes over the posterior roots of the occipital nerve—one on the side of the spine, the other an inch farther off—the relief was speedy, and the improvement lasted for many weeks.

For superficial pain, and to promote muscular activity, the induced or Faradic is more useful.

The pain of localized electro-magnetism curing the chronic pains of myalgia.—Mrs. ——, æt. 28, of a nervous temperament, and a feeble, ill-developed muscular system, consulted me in 1854. For eighteen months she had suffered from constant aching, wearing pains all over the back, shoulders, and sides. She had been under the care of a skilful doctor for a long time before coming to me, had taken tonics in abundance, and used many external applications without relief to the ceaseless distressing pains. I tried various medicines and applications, shower-baths, hot and cold douching, all to no purpose. She described her state as of a number of separate pains, as a distinct aching in many points all over the back, shoulders, and sides. The nearest analogue I could think of, was the peculiar pain which the application of Faradic electricity causes. For half an hour every other day for a month, I applied the electro-magnetic current with wet sponges over the seat of pain. It perfectly and permanently cured her.

In infantile paralysis the use of the constant continuous current is productive of much benefit; when it ceases to do good the induced current may be found to follow up the advantage.

CHAPTER XIII.

HYDROPATHY.

OF all the boons to humanity which the empirical method has conferred, the discovery of hydropathy by Priessnitz may be considered the greatest. Hydropathy in England took deep root at Malvern, where the purest water was associated with fresh air and lovely surroundings. In water-cure treatment immense improvement afterwards arose at Matlock Bank, where Mr. Smedley worked much good by hot-water fomentations, and warm spongings followed by cold douches, from which much better therapeutic results followed than from the old-fashioned cold-water cure. Many delicate ladies and young children who became exhausted under cold bathing were restored to health by the alternation of hot and cold.

In consulting practice in large towns, patients frequently seek the help of the physician that, experience soon shows him, cannot get well at home. The well-regulated treatment at the hydropathic establishment is often his best prescription. In Germany this is better understood. A patient of mine, travelling in the Tyrol, took a long journey to Vienna, to consult the celebrated Dr. Oppolzer, the leading physician in Austria. After examining the patient, he said, "I prescribe hydropathy as the most suitable treatment for your case." The doctor took his fee, and said no more than, "There is a good hydropathic establishment at ———." The patient at once followed the prescription with much benefit.

The wet sheet pack is a most valuable aid in the treatment of many diseases, especially of the skin and kidneys. After an hour's pack, the use of a quickly administered cold shallow-bath, followed by a brisk walk, has a very beneficial influence on chronic inaction of liver.

In diarrhœa the hot blanket pack is invaluable; the free perspiration it induces displaces the discharge from the gastric intestinal mucous membrane. In the worst cases of measles it has as good an action as the cold wet pack in scarlatina.

A person suffering from cold feet and languor of circulation finds a most pleasant sensation of warmth for many hours after a cold bath, and a sense of wretchedness and languor after a warm one.

The sitz-bath used for a short time—ten or twelve minutes—tends to draw blood from the deeper organs of the pelvis and abdomen to the skin; but if the use of the sitz bath be prolonged to an hour it has the opposite effect, and attracts blood to the hæmorrhoidal vessels, the uterus, ovaries, and bladder. It may cause piles to bleed, or increase the menstrual flow, cause the bladder to secrete more mucus, and thus relieve pain. It may relieve the congested lungs in bronchitis. In congestive headaches its effect is often magical, especially if a handkerchief wet with cold water is kept on the head during the bath.

The foot-bath often suits better than the sitz-bath in promoting the menstrual flow, and in the relief of nervous or congestive headache. In the latter case the addition of two ounces of mustard increases its efficacy.

The cold foot-bath has the happiest effect in curing cold feet. Ladies who suffer so much from cold feet at night find themselves miserably cold towards morning after a hot foot-bath; but the reactive warmth after a cold foot-bath lasts all night.

The shower-bath stimulates and freshens up the nervous centres and the superficial nerves. It seems to surprise or frighten the nervous system into good behavior for the day. The action of the shower-bath in the healthy causes a jerky, sudden, spasmodic act of breathing and of the muscles, exactly akin to spasms, convulsions, hysteria.

If the shower-bath is not convenient, the ordinary sponging or sitz-bath answers pretty well. Into the empty bath a pail of hot water is thrown, to sponge in for three or four minutes; a can or jug of cold water thrown into the hot cools it suddenly, or cold water left in a tub at the side of the bath may be used to sponge over the body after the warm.

The two-pail douche is a most useful and agreeable bath, easily arranged by the patient sitting in an empty bath, the can of cold being spouted immediately after the can of warm.

In cases of paralysis the plan advised by Dr. Brown-

Séquard is very effectual. The patient sitting on a board across a sitz-bath, the attendant flops the spine with flannels or sponges dipped in hot water for a minute, then with cold for a minute, and so on for ten or fifteen minutes once or twice a day. The douche-bath has an excellent effect in the treatment of asthma, chorea, epilepsy, vertigo, hysteria.

The cold douche is a most powerful weapon in the doctor's power, for good or evil. At Malvern the strong cold douches were used to a most injudicious extent, the duration being too often left to the discretion of the bathman and the patient, till the spine became numb and exhausted. The douches are much better managed abroad, as at Plombières, where from twenty to thirty minutes of rain-douches are kept up with a constant alternation, hot for three or four minutes, cold for a minute or two, so on for half an hour, with the greatest benefit even to delicate ladies. In spine paraplegia the cold douche is dangerous, and not half so useful or agreeable as the alternate hot and cold douche, the action of which is more akin to the vital processes of the healthy nervous system, which seems to be a succession of alternations rather than a repetition of one action.

The spirit-lamp or the vapor-bath has a most admirable effect in congestions of the kidneys, liver, or brain; especially when followed by hot and cold sponging, then a warm bed, or a brisk walk.

J., æt. 56, plethoric constitution, sanguine lymphatic temperament; suffered for some days from distressing vertigo, fulness of the head, extreme lassitude. A vapor-bath for fifteen minutes followed by the cold rain douche gave the most immediate relief, and used daily for some weeks perfectly restored what threatened to become a serious case of organic disease of brain.

In many diseases of children the half pack, or the abdominal bandage, has the most admirable effect. It calms the excitable brain and promotes sleep. It increases the natural secretions of the intestines, and does well what purgatives do badly. When used warm and covered with oiled silk or macintosh cloth over the chest it relieves bronchitis. It is cleaner and more effective than linseed-meal poultices.

The local ascending douche is of infinite service in leucorrhœa from relaxation. In congestive or inflammatory uterine diseases, much care is needed to use tepid, not cold, water.

A doctor at Ems insisted upon a lady, the patient of a friend, using the internal douche quite cold. It caused sudden and severe congestion of the ovaries, which lasted six weeks.

I sent a lady to a well-known hydropathic establishment in Yorkshire. For a slight degree of uterine relaxation (prolapsus) the doctor ordered her a daily cold-water vaginal douche. This caused permanent contraction of the vagina. Before the use of the cold douches a full-size Hodge's pessary fitted well and afforded perfect relief from the weight and bearing down. After a month's use of the cold douche even the smallest size could not be retained, and the vagina became permanently contracted.

15

The ascending douche is useful also in relaxed piles disposed to exhausting loss of blood.

When hydropathy seemed at a standstill it received a great impetus through the use of the thermometer, which has given precision to the use of cold baths. In typhoid fever especially hydropathy promises much. It is only suitable for the treatment of severe cases, and of dangerous complications. An ordinary uncomplicated case of typhoid does much better if sponging with tepid water all over the body three to four times a day is the sum total of water treatment.

At Basle, in October, 1869, I watched with great interest the experiments of Professor Liebermeister in the treatment of typhoid fever by means of nearly cold baths.

Believing that the increased elevation of temperature is the essential symptom of typhoid fever, the Professor keeps the patient in a full bath, at about 80° Fahr., for ten minutes, repeating it as often as the temperature rises beyond 102°.

I found the doctor at a quarter past eight in the laboratory of the hospital deeply engaged in experiments on the exhalation of carbonic acid from the body. The nurses take the temperature every two hours, marking it on the tablet over the head of the bed. In most, if not all, cases the bath seemed disagreeable to the patients; many make much noise as a protest, and even after having taken many baths still there is not much real liking for it. In answer to my question to one patient, a young man about twenty-five, who had taken fifty-six baths, he said, " I endured the bath, never liked it."

Wine is given after the bath, in bad cases brandy. The bath is repeated in some cases very often, even six or eight times in the day; as often as the temperature rises again.

Every patient on admission to the hospital gets one warm bath with soap, but soap is used in none of the cold baths. A full dose of calomel is given in most cases once, and if that does not purge, one or two doses more are given.

In the use of cold water in the treatment of disease Dr. Wilson Fox's cases mark an era of great importance, although the actual result of the application of cold is *mixed up with* the free use of brandy, yet few physicians would hesitate to adopt the cold-water treatment in diseases where the temperature reaches 107° or upwards.

In ordinary cases of fever, or acute diseases, it is far safer and easier to have the patient carefully sponged all over three or four times a day with warm water and soap. The patient and the friends often dread the wet-sheet pack, but do not object to the warm-water sponging; the latter is practicable with the help of one nurse. The former requires the doctor's constant presence and two or three additional nurses. The use of the cold bath to reduce the temperature in fever or acute rheumatism is a good illustration of Galen's law—"contraria contrariis curantur." The reaction after the cold bath, or cold pack, is towards the production of heat, hence the need of frequent repetition directly the temperature rises again.

"Cold water is no panacea for typhoid. It does not prevent death in a certain proportion of cases. Applied early, even during the first week, it does not cause the fever to abort. It often prevents the fever taking a severe course, limits the tendency to complications, especially the more dangerous ones, and makes the convalescence easier and more rapid. It moderates the mortality from typhoid. The chief effect of the bath is the lowering of temperature, which is largely due to the excitement of skin transpiration. If the skin be already perspiring, there is no need for the artificial cooling."*

The Turkish bath in disease of the lungs, especially in phthisis, works in compensation to the impeded lung function. It also stimulates appetite and the waste and repair of tissue, but like a keen double-edged sword it may cut the wrong way if not carefully handled.

In disease of the heart the Turkish bath often does harm, and seldom good. In organic disease of the liver it has a good palliative action. In that state called biliousness, deranged secretions of the stomach and duodenum, it relieves defective internal secretion by increased external. It is invaluable in such cases to those who cannot afford time or money for horse exercise. In diseases of the skin the use of the Turk-

---

* The Therapeutical Application of Cold Water in Febrile Diseases, by D. F. Kuchenmeister, Berlin.

ish bath is invaluable, and in acute and chronic catarrh of the mucous membrane of the nose, throat, and bronchial tubes. Amongst even the poor it is appreciated in such cases.

In many very severe and obstinate diseases of the nervous system, the use of the Turkish bath has an effect all but magical. It lessens the irritability and sense of miserable oppression, clears the head, and imparts buoyancy and freshness—that, too, when medicines, mild or strong, only exasperate and worry. The violent perspiration and the shampooing seem to lift a cloud, or take the tension off the nervous system. In a much less degree the same relief follows the use of the lamp-bath, followed by hot and cold sponging. In disease of the kidneys, the Turkish bath sets up a vigorous action on the skin, to supplement the imperfect action, and assist the excretion of urea and uric acid from the blood.

In acute and subacute diseases of the kidneys, much better results follow the use of the lamp- or vapor-bath, which can be used at bedtime, when a gentle continuous action is kept up all night in the warm bed; whereas, after the Turkish bath, much evil is done by the sudden reaction of cold washing and exposure to the cold air on returning home. I have been much discouraged with the imperfect results of the use of the Turkish bath in diseases of the kidneys, except in the rare circumstance of the patient living in the establishment where he takes his bath.

The action of the Turkish bath is curative according to the law of "similia similibus curantur."

Attacks of profuse perspiration, recurring for four years, cured by the Turkish bath:

Miss ——, æt. 55, living at Barnsbury. For four years confined to the bed or the bedroom by frequently-recurring heats, followed by profuse perspiration, lasting for twenty-four hours. The attacks were irregularly intermittent,—at times every third day, occasionally every day,—preceded by the most distressing throbbing in the head. The monthly periods continued regularly. She had been under the care of several medical practitioners without benefit. She had spent a large part of the four years in bed profusely perspiring. I advised the use of Turkish baths. The exertion of driving to and from the establishment proved so exhausting, that I urged her to leave her own home and go into the hydropathic establishment at Barnet, so as to take the Turkish bath daily without effort. The result exceeded my most sanguine expectations. In six weeks chills and perspiration ceased, and her life of sweating in bed every alternate day was exchanged for an active open-air life, out walking before breakfast, etc. The cure was perfect and permanent, and removed her altogether from the need of further medical treatment.

CHAPTER XIV.

FOOD.

"Such food as is most grateful, though not so wholesome, is to be preferred to that which is better but distasteful."—HIPPOCRATES.

"A pound of flesh is enormously superior to a pound of cabbage; yet to a rabbit the cabbage is the superior food, whilst to the dog it is no food at all."—G. H. LEWES's *Physiology of Common Life.*

IN the prescribing of food, knowledge of law affords much aid to the physician. In the management of children's diseases the doctor is beset by such a multitude of infant's foods, that it requires tact to keep to the food—milk—which nature has provided as exactly suited to the digestive organs, and capable of supplying all the materials for the growth of the various tissues of the body as well as for the life-work or functions of the organs.

Unless the mother's constitution is diseased, or her ancestors were subject to idiotcy or insanity, she ought to nurse her child, at least for a few months. With good management of diet, exercise, sleep, her milk ought to suit the child. Should it disagree, it may be for want of dilution, and the addition to the mother's drink of two or three pints of seltzer-water or thin barley-water may speedily improve its quality.

Of all the artificial foods, that of Liebig's is probably the best. Chapman's wheat-flour seems also to supply the materials—organic and inorganic—for the natural growth of the young tissues.

We should never swerve (except in the case of convulsions) from the first principle of diet in children. Without milk, or its equivalent, the child cannot prove healthy or strong in constitution.

To the constant reiteration that " milk does not agree with the child," the patience and skill of the doctor must give help to make it agree—by the addition of lime-water, if the curd forms too rapidly. In the opposite case of delay in its digestion, i. e., too slow coagulation, the addition of small quantities of pure pepsin wine has a very decided effect. Many cases of infants emaciated through diarrhœa I have seen thrive speedily on the addition of one-third of a teaspoonful of Bullock & Reynolds's pepsin wine to each bottle of milk. For children in the country the ordinary infusion of rennet, used by the farmers for making cheese, answers just as well.

With many infants the best food is fresh cream, mixed with twice as much hot water.

For the healthy development of children, parents ought to know that it is necessary to supply each child up to the age of twelve or fourteen with an abundant quantity of milk, irrespective of all other food. For those who can afford it, the allowance ought to be at least one to one and a half pints of milk to each child. It is far better to lessen the expenditure of tea, sugar, wine, beer, jam, pastry, and endure the sight of a heavy milk bill. Even in the families of the rich this is too often neglected. How often can the doctor trace this neglect in childhood to be the cause of deformed spines or of consumption later on.

For the management of a household, wise arrangements often prove less expensive and less troublesome than foolish. In the end much of the happiness and health of the family depends upon the *intelligence* shown in the selection of the food-supply.

To spend less upon farinaceous food and pastry, enables the poor householder to spend more on fresh vegetables, fruit, and milk. To have brown bread on the table as well as white causes no extra expense and prevents the necessity for purgative medicines.

With healthy young children it is far better to feed well and carefully, but not to give alcoholic stimulants except during the hot weather, when claret wine diluted with twice as much ice-water does infinite service; refreshing without stimulating, it tends to increase the appetite. Kept as medicine for the hot weather, it does not beget the desire for stimulants. Pure Bordeaux wine contains so little alcohol that it is more akin to an aromatic fruit juice, and becomes the antidote to intemperance. The opposite obtains with beer, the use of which in early years gives children a thirst for all stimulants.*

---

* When parents can afford to do so it is wise to give their children no wine except the finest, such as Chateau Lafitte or Margaux. The delicate flavor of such wines induces a dislike to all ordinary alcoholic fluid.

In childhood and youth waste and repair are alike active. The more abundant the supply of food the better—children will rarely eat too much good simple food. Not to interfere with this rapid growth, it is desirable to limit the use of tea and coffee. As occasional luxuries these are very good for children, but as regular daily beverages very injurious. As enabling the economy to use less food by limiting the natural waste, they are as unfit for children as they are most useful for adults—with whom want of appetite, anxiety, or poverty may lessen the supply of nourishment. With such the use of tea and coffee unquestionably exercises a powerful influence in lessening the need and enabling the organs to work with a smaller supply of food. So far it is an evil, but too often an unavoidable evil.

In advising food we should have the distinct principle before us to apportion the quantity and quality to the more or less rapid waste, and the work or functions of the body.

The diet of adults requires much more precaution amongst the rich and the well-to-do than amongst the poor, with whom quantity is apt to be deficient, and with whom hard labor tends to prevent the injurious effects of bad quality. Especially with those leading sedentary lives, excess in the quantity of food acts injuriously. It throws excessive work upon the various organs of life; the liver and kidneys especially, on which the task devolves of carrying out of the body the portions of food digested in the stomach, and not needed to supply the waste of tissue or to generate force.*

The teaching of Liebig did much to lead to the excessive use of animal food in England, which is so potent a cause in the production of gout and lithic acid gravel. Fortunately for humanity *most* of the excess of animal food is simply wasted. Dr. Parkes's experiments prove this very clearly; yet even a small portion of the excess is sufficient in the course of years to leave too much urea and uric acid in the system, especially when the decline of years finds the liver and kidneys unequal to the extra exertion of carrying it out of the system.

The Diet of Age.—Soon after fifty the tissues and organs of most human beings begin to show signs of the degeneration of age, the organic yielding gradually to the inorganic or chemical force, which inexorably asserts its predominance. The "arcus senilis" too often tells a tale as to the increasing hardness of the coats of the arteries, which gradually lose their elasticity and become more fragile. The bones, muscles, tendons, joints also became more stiff and unyielding, and the shape of the body alters from the gradual yielding of the spine. As age comes on it is desirable to lessen the supply of food rich in nitrogen and inorganic constituents, so as to keep the tissues from absorbing an excess of chemical elements; also to relieve the stomach

* " Excess of nutriment, or change in conditions of life in the parent forms, *causes variability*, which, however, is frequently not manifested for several generations."—Darwin on Variation of Animals and Plants.

and glands from overwork, and spare the kidneys from the strain of excreting the excess of urea and uric acid, which, blocking up the tubuli uriniferi, may lead to granular degeneration and albuminuria.

Diet in Exhaustion or Disease of the Nervous System : Neuralgia, Epilepsy, Paralysis.—The proportion of oily matter in the brain and spine and the ganglia of the sympathetic is enormously in excess of that in any other organ of the body in health. Hence the need of an abundant supply of fat, oil, butter, and cream, in most diseases of the nervous system, including neuralgia, epilepsy, and paralysis. Thus it is also that an abundant supply of fresh meat is so relished by literary men, and those who undergo sustained mental exertion ; even the so-called lean of beef contains much fat spread out in layers through the muscular fibres ; thus a plentiful supply of oily matter is taken unawares. Alcoholic fluids in moderation prove most useful in all exhausting diseases of the nervous system, but if taken in excess become the fruitful cause of organic disease of the brain.

Hæmorrhage.—It is in severe floodings, especially during or after confinement, that the effects of brandy or wine seem most marvellous. At such times there seems to be a capacity for absorbing and utilizing quantities of alcohol which to the same individual in health would prove semi-poisonous, and cause actual intoxication. To arrest such deadly hæmorrhage an imperial pint of brandy has often been given in a few hours without the slightest disturbance of the sensorium.

Well may the physician in such cases trust to experience, and disown all arguments against alcohol.

In disease of the stomach it is of great consequence to prescribe food that is light and not irritating. In many such cases the patient will gain strength upon fish, fowl, and light custard puddings, when a more generous diet only creates misery and suffering. In disease of the intestines this is even more needful, the stomach digestion may be good and the intestinal bad. Here small quantities of soft meats, such as boiled neck of mutton, stewed chicken, boiled rice, become so thoroughly digested in the stomach as to cause very little *débris* to enter the intestines.

In 1860 I attended a lady in Euston Square, aged 82, for an attack of gastric fever, characterized by excessive dryness of the mouth, with yellowish fur on tongue, heat of skin, constipation, restless nights, and exhaustion. It proved a very tedious attack, although dieted as we thought carefully with beef tea, milk, brandy and water, etc. Relapse after relapse occurred, but at length she recovered in seven weeks. A year afterwards she had another attack, precisely similar, but from the first I prescribed no food but sugar and water and brandy. She made an excellent recovery in three weeks, and got well in less than half the time of the attack the previous year. Weak beef tea was given her two or three times during this attack, and within three hours each time there was such a marked increase of fever, that the friends were perfectly convinced that it was best to confine her diet to sugar and water and brandy. Some months afterwards she went to Liverpool, and after a time had another attack of the same gastric fever, for which the local doctor fed her well, as he said, but relapse after relapse occurred, and she died of exhaustion in seven weeks.*

Careful Dieting in Organic Disease of Stomach.—In 1866 I attended a most instructive case, in Highbury New Park—a gentleman aged 68, suffering for a year from malignant disease of the stomach. He had been attended for some time by a general practitioner in the neighborhood, and a London physician of eminence. They agreed upon the incurable nature of his disease, and prescribed dilute nitro-hydrochloric acid. Every dose only aggravated his suffering, and, in the words of the patient, seemed to tear his inside. Getting rapidly emaciated he sent for me. He suffered from constant burning pain with soreness all over the epigastric region, where a solid, hard, non-pulsating tumor afforded but too positive evidence of the nature of his disease, which caused incessant nausea and frequent vomiting of grumous brownish fluid, containing broken-down blood-particles. I gave a most unfavorable prognosis and prescribed sulphate of atropia $\frac{1}{100}$th of a grain, *i. e.*, ten drops of the third decimal dilution, three times a day, half an hour before meals. His diet was limited to calves' head, boiled sole, oysters, jelly, bread puddings, and milk. In two days I visited him again, and was delighted to find pain and sickness gone, and the patient

---

* At the same time in the same house I was in attendance upon her grandson, aged six, for scrofulous disease of the hip-joint. For him I prescribed butcher's meat and Bass's ale three times a day. He made a good and perfect recovery.

expressing the greatest relish for his diet. Week after
week for two months he kept on improving, gained flesh
to a surprising extent, took much open-air exercise, and
kept free from pain and sickness. To his family I was
obliged to say again and again," It is only a temporary
improvement ; the disease is of an incurable nature."
They hinted that I was over-cautious, till the end of two
months, when all the bad symptoms slowly advanced
again ; and although pain and suffering were mitigated,
death slowly came.

CHAPTER XV.

CONCLUSION.

"THAT is the divinest faculty of the human mind that sees law in the most minute as in the greatest actions." * "For does not science tell us that its highest striving is after the ascertainment of a unity, which shall bind the smallest things with the greatest?"† All progress in knowledge lies in the direction of simplicity and exactness. The study of natural forces has led to the discovery of the interdependence and correlation of all those forces. In this grand field of investigation in physical science, a large and most important share has been taken by medical men. Dr. Bence Jones, in England, and Dr. Meyer, in Germany, are good illustrations that the practice of medicine is not incompatible with the pursuit of physical science.

Accustomed to work under exact laws in physical and physiological science, how strange that, when the physician passes into the field of therapeutics, he is too often satisfied to grope in the dark with arbitrary rules in the treatment of disease !

The most important investigation in therapeutics now is to search for the laws of action of medicinal

---

* Professor Tyndall.   † The Mill on the Floss.

agents, and discover what relationship the action of
curative agents in disease holds to their action on the
healthy human body. Not that the science of therapeutics is to become an abstract problem in mathemat-
ics, but that the physician should be guided by accurate knowledge of natural laws in health and disease.
Then, indeed, medical science becomes like what the
philosophy of Bacon was said to be compared to the
Greek philosophy—"as a vineyard or an olive-ground
bearing abundant refreshment and fruit for humanity,
not the intricate wood of briers and thistles, from which
those who lost themselves in it brought back many
scratches but no food."

In the very attractive field of experimental and
microscopic investigation of the nervous system, we
must be careful not to put our interpretations on the
facts, which should be allowed to speak for themselves.
The more we become acquainted with the ultimate
action of medicines, the more essential it is not to for-
sake the reign of law which brings the ordinary into
harmony with the ultimate or finer action, in the search
for which we must not let the more delicate actions hide
those recognizable by ordinary modes of observation.
The most careful observation of the action of medicines
in disease, proves that in most cases there is a distinct
relationship between that action and the effects of the
same medicine on the human body in health. The
relationship may be that of similarity or of antagonism;
but there it is, and *cannot be overlooked* but to the det-
riment of the human family and of medical science.

It may be said that laws of therapeutics may yet be

discovered not having any relationship between the action of medicinal agents on the human body in health and in disease. To this it may be answered, all discovery in science has been in the direction of unity and of simplicity; primary laws include secondary, and all harmonize. No discovery can contradict truth; its foundations may be shaken but not removed.

The correlation of organic forces is as true as that of the inorganic. Remedial action in disease must ever have a scientific and practical relationship to the natural force in health. Doubtless, there will ever be a large field for empirical medicine; genius often overleaps the boundaries of science when the latter degenerates into routine or safe orthodoxy. When strict theorists and dogmatists give an uncertain sound, it needs a dash of empiricism to cast aside conflicting theories and arrive at truth by insight. Whilst investigators and microscopists are working in the elucidation of the etiology and pathology of cholera, it is well for practical medicine that the instinct of genius should lead Niemeyer to the conclusion that there " is one clinical symptom of the most guiding value, the diarrhœa; and one pathological fact proved, viz., the intestinal lesion; and only one sort of treatment, the empiric management of this intestinal catarrh." In the early stage of not very severe diarrhœa, he gave a few doses of laudanum, but if the amendment was not rapidly perceptible, he abandoned the opium and had recourse to calomel (a grain every half hour) and *cold* wet packing. The cold packing especially relieved the sickness, so much so that patients cried out for the renewal of the cold as soon as the bandages became at all warm; * thus finding the harmony of the law of similars in prescribing for catarrhal flux of the intestines the medicine calomel, which has most power to cause flux of the same surface, and for the deadly coldness of collapse the ice-cold water applications.

The empirical method has been a favorite one in all ages, and has found its ablest and latest expounder in the great Niemeyer.

"Of late years medical explorers have recognized the only path by which therapeutic science can be advanced, and have followed it with brilliant results.

"Experiments made with medicaments upon the lower animals or upon healthy human beings, with all their scientific value, have as yet been of no direct service to our means of treating disease, and a continuation of such experiments give no prospect of such service .... nor would pathological investigation promote therapeutic success, unless directed more in accordance with the requirements of general medicine than has been done hitherto. The empirical method of investigating is the only rational and proper one for the study of therapeutics, or of any other department of natural science.

"The valuable labors, now under prosecution in this long-neglected field of treatment of disease, by means of which already the value of certain important articles hitherto ill-appreciated has been accurately determined, have received general recognition, and thus a final blow has been given to the dominion of disheartening therapeutical nihilism. This success, as an example of which I will merely mention the discovery of the antipyretic action of quinine in typhus, pneumonia, etc., and the establishment of precise indications for the use of digitalis in disease of the heart, has caused the zeal for therapeutic experimentalism to assume a direction destined to lead to great

* Niemeyer on the "Symptomatic Treatment of Cholera," Practitioner, July 12th, pp. 40, 41.

results. Rightly supposing that even the rude experience of the
ignorant laity and their belief in the all-healing power of the
'cold-water cure' and the 'bread cure' have some foundation
in fact, the effect both of hydropathic treatment and that of the
continued limitation of the supply of water to the system have
been subject to rigid analysis. Such laudable abnegatism of
sectarian pride has been richly rewarded."*

Many thinkers and many great physicians have ad-
vocated the empirical method, yet it must be confessed
that the amount of tribute it has rendered to practical
medicine is small. It is fruitful and progressive only
when sustained by law, although not overtly recognized, yet in the main upholding it. Thus laws of
therapeutics reign and teach empirical medicine how
to extend its dominion. Without the backbone of
scientific principle, the empirical method fails. When
every doctor does only what is good in his own eyes,
empirical skill only leads to chaos and confusion; the
opinions of one man and of one age ruthlessly being
tossed aside by the next.

The great object of science in medicine is to enable
the doctor to have all his knowledge in hand to use
promptly and effectually for the individual sick person;
the facts of health, of disease, and of therapeutics, combined into leading principles that guide to a perfect
method of cure; the gathered up experience of years,
easily come at through law and order.

No doubt empirical medicine has conferred many rich
gifts upon the science and art of medicine. None more

* Niemeyer's Practical Medicine. Seventh German edition,
American translation.

valuable than the discovery of cinchona bark and of quinine, the usefulness of iodide of potassium in tertiary syphilis, and that of bromide of potassium in epilepsy. The use of cod-liver oil, of pepsin, pancreatin, ox-gall, etc.

The *Talmud:* " The day is short and the work is great; but the laborers are idle, though the reward be great and the master of the work presses."

" Law rules all things," cries the father of medicine. Truly, for the physician it is all things—evolution, development, nutrition, function, health, disease, treatment. Every addition to knowledge tells how essential for the true artist to have a deep substratum of unfailing science. Medical art, and the physician's skill, must have deep streams of unerring law to feed their growth, or they soon get dry and barren. The time is near when the highest tribute to the man will be, " He is a truly scientific physician;" now, it is often a byword for contempt. To silence that cry, it is for the man of science to cultivate the art of medicine till the perfect master's hand is known by perfect work. The truest and highest service allowed of God to His children is to serve one another.

It is not long ago since the practical man despised all books and reading. Such practical men quickly exposed their ignorance and helplessness in every obscure and difficult case. The just reproach, in the present age, for any physician is to have allowed science to pass by without gathering up its rich fruit. Truly it requires watchfulness and dexterity to know everything

that may conduce to the welfare of those intrusted to
our care.

In conclusion, "as a fellow-laborer in one great common work bearing upon the highest interests of humanity," I search out for myself what I desire to make
known to others—every aid for the sick and suffering
that science and art can give to the physician, taking at
their true value all laws and principles of healing, and
using them for the elaboration and perfecting of the
art of medicine; so that I may be a workman approved
of my Master, and a servant fit to minister amongst the
sick, the sorrowful, and the weak.

APPENDIX.

—

A Grand Field for Empirical Science.—Certain diseases, like cancer, defy the science and art of medicine and surgery to do more than alleviate suffering. Yet the man of science should not despair of finding curative means to arrest that terrible disease. The subcutaneous injection of medicine affords the most likely means of reaching its source and its cause. Watching the gradual infiltration of the tissues by the delicate microscopic cancer-cells, it would seem that the track or line of infection of the constitution from the earliest stage of scirrhus seems to be through the delicate structure of the cellular tissue and the intercellular spaces.

What a boon to suffering humanity if any chemical agent could be found to follow this dire infection of the constitution, and leave the nodule of scirrhus to shrivel and die, without retaining its power to destroy the life of the tissues! Our search for agents to neutralize or destroy the cancer disease should lie in the direction of those which shut it up—as it were encase these microscopic cells, and coagulate or harden the intercellular fluid. The best of such is chromic acid, which in the field of the microscope is seen, even in a solution as dilute as one part in one thousand of water, speedily to define, as if dissecting out, the delicate cells, hardening and inclosing the nuclei, closing up their walls, thus preventing the diffusion of their contents. A solution of chromic acid as weak as one part in one thousand of water, wastes its chief strength on the tissues, and leaves little for absorption. Osmic acid is still more potent to harden the cells, but it is a stronger poison to the system generally.

Professor Billroth's use of arsenic internally, and by subcutaneous injection in lymphoma, gives encouragement to the trial of the same in true scirrhus. In malignant lymphoma he gives, with the most marked success, Fowler's solution morning and evening, after food, in doses gradually increasing from five to twenty drops. Also two or three times a day a subcutaneous injection of a few drops of Fowler's solution into the parenchymatous structure of the glands.*

Dr. Broadbent's suggestion of dilute acetic acid subcutaneously injected, failed from its being the opposite in action to chromic acid, as it dissolves the cell-walls, sets the nuclei free to flood the intercellular spaces with a rapidly infecting material that spreads through every allied organ and gland till the deadly constitutional cachexia is fully established.

Akin to the action of the subcutaneous injection, the use of chloroform in external applications bids fair to be useful in the treatment of external cancer. It is a most useful " carrier" to vegetable alkaloids, promoting

---

* The Practitioner, March, 1878, p. 213.

their absorption. Its action in causing the absorption of vegetable alkaloids seems to depend upon the removal of the cuticle, thus exposing the absorbing surface of the cutis vera. By long-continued use it might also cause mineral substances to pass into the tissues.

Of all diseases, the diagnosis of external cancer is the most easy. The sufferers from that disease should generally consult the surgeon or physician in its earliest stage; then careful trial of the subcutaneous injection might be commenced in the scirrhous nodule itself, or all around it, so as to inject all the gland-structure and the intercellular spaces; thus, if possible, to shut up, as if in a case, the prolific structure. To insure accuracy of treatment, use should be made of a large syringe, even to the size of half an ounce, with a very dilute solution, or else the ordinary fifteen-minim injection repeated several times all round the circumference of the tumor, till every avenue of infective absorption is shut up.

In an extensive practice during thirty years, with a large number of unsuccessful cases, I have been three times encouraged as to the possibility of curing cancer.

Mrs. ———, a thin, delicate-looking lady, aged 44, consulted me for a profuse putrid discharge from the womb that had existed for many months, causing emaciation and loss of strength. Her own doctor, having treated her unsuccessfully for some time, took her to Dr. ———, a well-known specialist in Grosvenor Street, who pronounced her to be suffering from cancer uteri, and prescribed palliative treatment, which

17

proved useless. Subsequently she placed herself under my care.

On examination I found a large dark-colored, irregular fungous growth, protruding from the os uteri, a well-marked instance of the true cauliflower excrescence. For six weeks, through the speculum, I touched the surface daily with arsenic powder,—one part arsenious acid to nine of white sugar,—at the same time administering one-thirtieth of a grain of arsenious acid (three drops of the first centesimal dilution) three times a day. At the end of the fifth week the entire mass slowly broke down and came away. At the end of the sixth week a perfectly healthy surface was left, all the profuse, foul-smelling discharge ceased, and she recovered health and strength. For twelve years she continued in perfect health, till this year (1877), when evidence of scirrhus of the stomach has shown itself.

About five years ago, a lady from the midland counties, aged 44, consulted me. I found a hard, irregular nodule of scirrhus in the breast, with retraction of the nipple, two or three small glands in the axilla enlarged. She was in low health, thin, sallow-looking—in every way a most unfavorable case. The family doctor pronounced the disease to be cancer. She then came to London to consult me. The case seemed to me to be well-marked scirrhus in the early stage. After examining her, I sent her to Mr. Thomas Nunn, whom I knew to have a large experience of cancer at the Middlesex Hospital. He examined her most carefully, and sent her back to me with a note that, in his opinion, the case was one of unmistakable scirrhus, specially drawing my attention to the well-marked retraction of the nipple. He considered the case an unsuitable one for operation.

As the last resource, not to give up the case as hopeless, I then prescribed a strong lotion of hydrastis canadensis, two ounces of the strong undiluted tincture mixed with two drachms of chloroform, applied night and day, freely sprinkled upon lint covered with oil-silk. Also the internal use of seven drops of the pure tincture of hydrastis canadensis three times a day. The lady returned to her home, and carried out the treatment steadily for six weeks. She then wrote to me that she was so much better that her family doctor was much surprised at the change. Soon afterwards she came to London to see me, and I was equally surprised, as the disease had nearly disappeared. I sent her again to Mr. Nunn, who, comparing his notes of the case as it was two months before, was quite taken aback. The improvement continued, and although five years have elapsed since, there has been no return of the disease, and the lady continues in perfect health.

In this case the disease may not have been true cancer; yet it lacked no characteristic of that disease. Mr. Nunn, the country doctor, and I agreed that it seemed a well-marked case of scirrhus in the early stage. The result of the treatment was most satisfactory and palpable.

Mrs. S——, aged 57, consulted me in 1875 for a hard, irregular enlargement of the left breast; the nipple retracted, and the glands in the left axilla en-

larged and rather painful.   Her mother had died of
cancer of the tongue.   I prescribed a paste of hydrastis
canadensis :

Pulv. hydrastis,	· ℥j
Glyc. Amyli, .	· ℥ij
Chloroformyl,	· ℥j

The application of the paste brought out a copious
pustular eruption all round the breast.   This caused
the swelling and hardness to lessen ; gradually the enlargement in the axilla passed off, and the breast became
soft.   She continued the application of the paste for
two years, till nearly all trace of the original disease
disappeared, although the nipple is still slightly retracted.

www.ingramcontent.com/pod-product-compliance
Lightning Source LLC
Chambersburg PA
CBHW021801190326
41518CB00007B/401